Candida Cookbook for Beginners

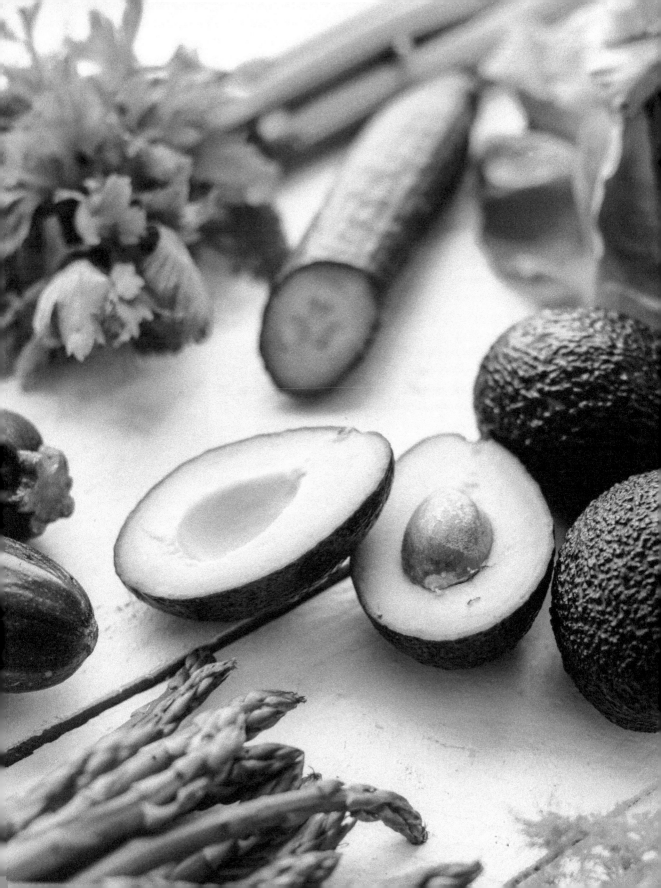

Candida Cookbook
for Beginners

85 Recipes to Alleviate Symptoms and Restore Gut Health

Sondi Bruner, CNP

ROCKRIDGE
PRESS

Interior and Cover Designer: Scott Petrower
Art Producer: Samantha Ulban
Editor: Claire Yee

Photography © 2021 Annie Martin, Cover; Stocksy / Ina Peters, p. ii; Stocksy / Pixel Stories, p. v; Stocksy / RENÁTA DOBRÁNSKA, p. vi; Stocksy / Alberto Bogo, p. x; Stocksy / Laura Adani, p. 18; Stocksy / Ina Peters, p. 23; StockFood / Keller & Keller Photography, pp. 31, 118; StockFood / Harley, Victoria, p. 39; Stocksy / Harald Walker, pp. 46, 51; Stocksy / Pixel Stories, p. 62; StockFood / Winkelmann, Bernhard, p. 67; Stocksy / Davide Illini, p. 75; StockFood/Greg Vore, p. 83; StockFood / DeA Picture Library, p. 90; StockFood / Kirchherr, Jo, p. 94; iStock, p. 106; Stocksy / Jeff Wasserman, p. 125; StockFood / Janssen, Valerie, p. 126.

ISBN: Print 978-1-64876-973-3 | eBook 978-1-64876-281-9
R0

To my kindred sweet tooth spirits:
You can step away
from that bag of chocolate chips
and still love life.

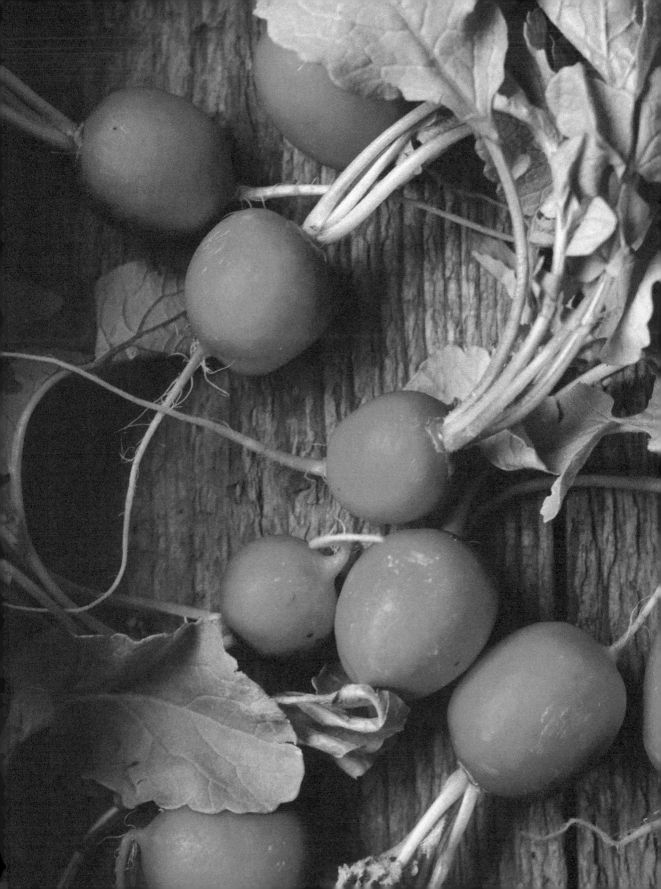

Contents

Introduction

I was diagnosed with an inflammatory bowel disease at 18 years old. And throughout my young adulthood, I thought I knew everything there was to know about how my condition affected my body—from the Western medical perspective, anyway.

At 26, after years of scoffing at natural health treatments, I found myself in the office of a naturopathic doctor. I was bloated all the time, felt sick every time I ate, could barely focus, was too tired to exercise, and had constant diarrhea—even in the middle of the night. My gastroenterologist had essentially told me there was nothing he could do for me, so I needed to explore other options.

Being the know-it-all I was, as I sat across from the naturopath, I assumed she would confirm what I already recognized—that Crohn's disease was the root of my problems—and then she would lay out an alternative plan to address it. So imagine my surprise when she told me she suspected my current situation was caused by candida, a freeloading fungus that can invade the body and produce a multitude of health issues. I had never heard of candida and was somewhat doubtful, but I was willing to try her protocol of antifungals, homeopathic remedies, and a strict candida-free diet.

In hindsight, I realize her assessment was perfectly logical. Yes, I had a digestive disorder that compromised my immune system and disrupted my gut flora—two prime factors that can create a ripe environment for candida to thrive. I was also addicted to sugary foods (I even compulsively ate cookies or ice cream for breakfast, even though I didn't really want them—it was like someone else was controlling that ice cream scoop). I was on the birth control pill. I had recently taken multiple rounds of antibiotics. I ate junk—we're talking food from boxes and cans and bottles. When all these factors combined with my existing health condition, it's no wonder candida threw a party in my gut.

I didn't know it at the time, but that visit and candida diagnosis would set me on the path to better health, culinary prowess, and even a new career. The candida-free diet was very strict: no sugar, no yeast, no alcohol, no wheat, no processed foods, no chocolate, no fruit, and more, which was especially challenging for me because I didn't know how to cook! I had to toss out everything I thought I knew—along with basically everything in my refrigerator and pantry—and start afresh.

Many years later, I left my career in communications to study holistic nutrition. I had learned firsthand about the powerful impact foods have on our health, and I wanted to share that knowledge with others and help them get better, too.

Now I specialize in digestive health and allergy-friendly diets, focusing on menu planning and recipe development in order to give people like you the ease and power to facilitate your own wellness.

A candida-free diet and a step-by-step action plan offer the structure and tools you need to oust candida from your system, improve your digestion, support the liver, and nourish the friendly bacteria in your gut. The heart of this book, and what I'd like you to focus your effort and attention on, is Phase 1: Repair. It's the *candida detox* and—I'm not going to lie—it's the toughest part of the diet. Candida does not leave willingly or politely. It yells and clings to the doorframe.

There is a solution, and it can be found on your plate. In this book, you'll discover a number of tools to aid you on your journey to a candida-free life: information about common candida causes and symptoms, what foods to eat and avoid, how to incorporate probiotics, and 85 delicious recipes to support you on your journey. (The last part is my favorite!)

With these tools in hand, you'll be well on your way to fighting the symptoms that plague you and setting yourself on the path to better health—without candida along for the ride.

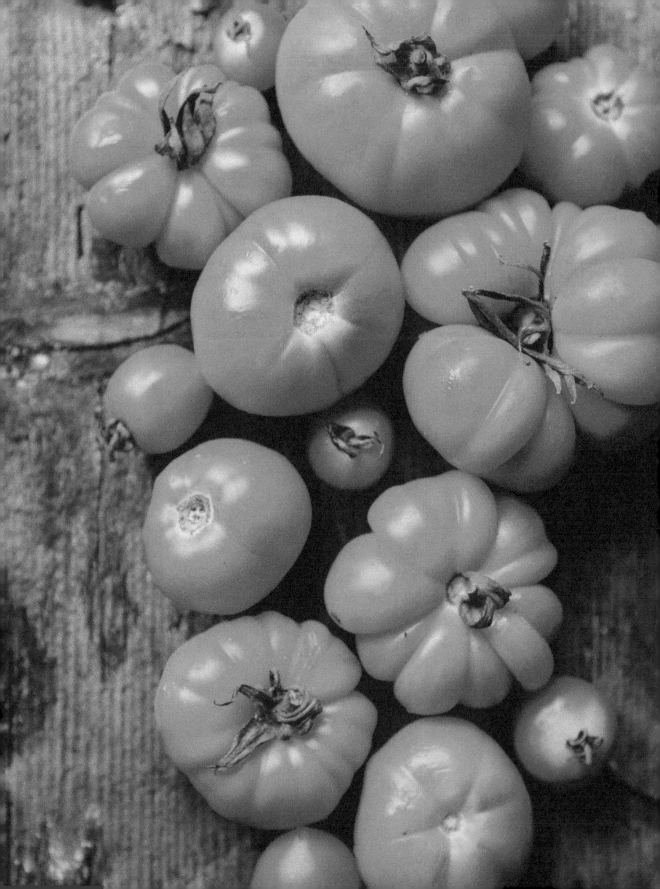

Chapter 1

A Beginner's Guide to the Candida-Free Diet

If you've heard of candida, it's likely you've learned to associate it with yeast infections in women. But contrary to popular belief, candida is a condition that can affect men, women, and children and can cause a variety of symptoms throughout multiple body systems. In fact, candida is linked to such a wide number of issues that it's often referred to as "candida-related complex" (CRC). In this chapter, we'll review what candida is, along with its symptoms, causes, and how to address it through dietary changes.

What Is Candida?

Our bodies contain a multitude of bacteria. In the digestive tract, there are hundreds of different species of bacteria that live with one another—sometimes everyone gets along and sometimes they don't.

One type of microorganism living in our bodies is a yeast-like fungus called *Candida albicans*, or candida, and it's found in our mouth, digestive tract, urinary tract, and on our skin. In normal amounts, candida lives harmoniously with other bacteria in the gut and is controlled by healthy digestive flora. But when the good microbes decrease or are destroyed, candida can go wild and take over, like dandelions you can't get rid of or ivy that threatens to overwhelm your flower beds.

When candida grows irrepressibly, it latches on to the lining of the intestinal tract and, like other parasites, begins to steal nutrients. As candida takes over, it activates cravings—particularly for sugary foods—so it can consume what it needs to proliferate. Eventually, candida can burrow through the intestinal lining and into the bloodstream, where it can cause further infection in the body. Some candida infections can be serious and even life threatening. The Centers for Disease Control and Prevention (CDC) estimates there 25,000 cases of invasive candidiasis every year.

Even worse, when candida conquers the digestive tract and feeds off its nutrients, it produces toxic by-products that spread in our bodies and can increase candida's negative impact on our health.

Candida-related complex can present in a wide variety of ways. Common symptoms include digestive upset, bloating, brain fog, itchiness, rashes, fatigue, joint pain, headaches, and food cravings, but that's not all. Dr. Warren Levin, author of *Beyond the Yeast Connection*, notes the following symptoms and conditions that can also be linked to candida:

- Acne
- Asthma
- Attention deficit hyperactivity disorder (ADHD)
- Autism
- Constant hunger
- Cradle cap
- Depression
- Eczema
- Endometriosis
- Gas
- Hay fever
- High/low blood pressure
- Hyperactivity
- Infertility
- Interstitial cystitis
- Irritability
- Kidney stones
- Low libido
- Lupus
- Polycystic ovary syndrome (PCOS)
- Premenstrual syndrome (PMS)
- Rheumatoid arthritis
- Schizophrenia
- Thyroiditis
- Urinary tract infections (UTIs)

Many questionnaires are available online that can help you establish whether you have candida (see Resources, page 128). This can be a good starting point, but be sure to work with a health-care practitioner to confirm the diagnosis.

The conventional medical community recognizes candida as an acute fungal infection: for example, a yeast infection, thrush (candida in the mouth), or invasive candidiasis. But the notion that candida is a widespread ailment connected to a multitude of organ systems is met with skepticism by some medical doctors or even considered a "fake" diagnosis by others. Fortunately, there are some Western physicians who take a broader view of candida beyond the acute or critical situation.

There is a plethora of alternative health-care practitioners such as naturopathic doctors, nutritionists, and functional medicine specialists who will listen to your concerns and work with you to improve your symptoms. It's important to find a practitioner you trust when dealing with candida.

Common Causes of Candida

Candida can proliferate for a variety of reasons and, often, it's not just a single thing that influences its growth. My experience with Crohn's disease left me with impaired digestion, a suppressed immune system, and intestinal dysbiosis (a microbial imbalance in my gut). Those facts alone left me at risk for developing candida, but I was also on birth control pills, had recently taken several rounds of antibiotics, and had a poor diet. Following, I'll review some common causes of candida in more detail so you can see how they operate.

Diet

Candida is an organism that feeds on sugar—particularly the white, refined kind. The typical North American diet is packed with sugars and refined carbohydrates, like white rice, bread, potatoes, and processed foods. These all spike blood sugar levels and flood our systems with the sweet stuff that makes candida sing. This sugar boost also comes with a decrease in immunity (sugar depresses the immune system).

Processed foods, chemicals, and aggravating food allergens also contribute to nutrient deficiencies, dysbiosis, the growth of candida, and a weak intestinal barrier, which can lead to leaky gut syndrome (see more on page 5). When dealing with candida, an important first step is addressing the diet, something we'll delve into later in much more detail.

Antibiotics

In certain situations, antibiotics are lifesaving and necessary. However, in the past few decades, they have been overprescribed, leading to a worldwide problem of antibiotic resistance, which means these drugs are becoming ineffective at treating serious illnesses.

Our digestive tract is home to a multitude of bacteria, both friendly and antagonistic. The problem with antibiotics is that they don't discriminate between the good bacteria and the bad bacteria—they wipe out *everything*. According to the *Encyclopedia of Natural Medicine*, antibiotic use is the most significant factor in developing candida, since antibiotics eliminate the healthy bacteria that keep candida in check. Remember, candida is extremely opportunistic; the second it has the chance to dominate the gut, it will.

This isn't to say that you should not take antibiotics if you need them. The key is to take them when it's essential for treating bacterial infections (antibiotics don't treat viruses like the pesky common cold). It's also helpful to follow a round of antibiotics with gut-boosting probiotics.

Stress

Stress impairs the immune system, which leaves us more vulnerable to infections that can influence candida's progression (plus, candida produces its own toxins that our antibodies must respond to, leaving the immune system overburdened).

Our stress response is regulated by the adrenal glands, and, when we're feeling stressed, the adrenals burn through our stores of magnesium—the "spark plug" for our adrenal glands. The stress hormone cortisol helps manage blood sugar levels, and tired adrenals don't produce as much cortisol, leaving excess sugar in the bloodstream for candida to feed on.

The (Contraceptive) Pill

The birth control pill pumps artificial hormones into the body and can lead to estrogen dominance, which can trigger the growth and breeding of candida. In one study (see References, page 132, U. of M. 2006), the use of oral contraceptives doubled the risk of developing a yeast infection. In addition, candida produces a waste product that mimics estrogen, tricking the body into believing there is more estrogen present.

Birth control use also strips the body of certain nutrients, such as B vitamins, zinc, and magnesium. Nutrient depletion can lead to dysbiosis, which can in turn cause your gut to spring a leak.

What Is Leaky Gut Syndrome?

Before diving into the common symptoms associated with candida, let's pause for a minute to focus on leaky gut syndrome, a gastrointestinal disorder that is believed to be closely linked to this condition. Our digestive tract has a specialized lining that allows beneficial nutrients to pass through it while blocking out harmful toxins, foreign substances, or large, undigested food particles. When our guts are strong and healthy, this barrier works efficiently to support and protect us. But when our intestinal lining isn't working properly, it develops holes that allow bacteria, bits of food, and toxins to pass through and into the bloodstream.

When those molecules burst through into the bloodstream where they're not supposed to be, the immune system springs into action, sending antibodies and cytokines (secreted by the immune system) to clean up the mess—which may just lead to further inflammation. This is called leaky gut syndrome, or intestinal permeability, and it can set the stage for a number of health problems, including:

- Aches and pains
- Acne
- Allergies
- Anxiety
- Arthritis
- Bloating
- Diarrhea
- Fatigue
- Food intolerances
- Mood swings
- Poor memory
- Rashes and hives

Leaky gut syndrome is influenced by a variety of factors, such as diet, stress, infection, dysbiosis (imbalance of microbes), drugs, nutrient deficiencies, environmental toxins, allergic reactions, and poor digestion.

What does all of this have to do with candida? Well, when candida grows out of control and grabs on to the gastrointestinal lining, it can punch holes in the gut that allow toxins to flow into the bloodstream and throughout the body. To tighten up that intestinal barrier, we need to heal the gut.

Diabetes

Diabetes occurs when the body doesn't produce enough insulin, or can't effectively use the insulin it creates, leading to an increase in sugar in the blood. As we already know, candida thrives on sugar, and the increase in sugar availability means there is more food for the candida to feed on. Studies show that diabetics are at an increased risk of developing candida.

Symptoms of Candida

The symptoms of candida-related complex can be far-reaching and numerous. Sometimes, it can be tricky to establish whether candida is the source, since it masquerades as many different ailments. For me, the digestive symptoms were frequent and troublesome. Most days, I was so bloated that I couldn't button or zip my pants, particularly by the end of the day. My diarrhea plagued me day and night. My appetite was nonexistent, except I always managed to eat bagels, ice cream, cookies, and candy.

Let's learn more about some common symptoms of candida so you'll know what to look for.

Physical

Candida loves warm, moist places, and the parts of our bodies that fit this bill are prime real estate for candida. Some physical symptoms candida sufferers might experience include:

Thrush. Oral candidiasis includes white spots in the mouth and on the tongue, redness, a sore throat, or cracked lips.

Urinary Tract Infections (UTIs) or Yeast Infections. UTIs occur when bacteria move into the urinary tract and cause infection and inflammation; if left untreated, a UTI can lead to a yeast infection. Vaginal yeast infections involve pain and soreness in the genitals, itching, a cottage cheese–like discharge, and pain during sex.

Invasive Candidiasis. This is common in hospitalized patients, and symptoms can include fever and chills that don't disappear after antibiotic treatment.

Diaper Rash. A soiled diaper is a perfect warm breeding ground for candida, leading to rashes in the skin creases, thighs, and on the genitals.

Other. Other physical symptoms that might appear are acne, itchiness, and hair, nail, and toe infections.

One challenge with the physical symptoms of candida is they are often treated with antibiotics, and once all the bacteria including the healthy ones in the gut are wiped out, we're left more susceptible to candida overgrowth.

Mental

As you've learned, candida generates waste by-products that circulate throughout the body, including the brain and nervous system. One of these by-products, acetaldehyde, is a neurotoxin that can lead to brain fog, nausea, and headaches—in some ways, similar to suffering from a hangover.

Also, excess consumption of sugar and refined carbohydrates can cause our blood sugar levels to spike, leading to bursts of energy followed by crashes, as well as mood swings and irritability. The primary mental symptoms of candida are:

- Brain fog
- Depression
- Fatigue
- Feeling "spaced out"
- Headaches
- Irritability
- Lack of focus or concentration
- Mood swings
- Nausea
- Poor memory

Digestive

Since so many bacteria live in the digestive tract (a whopping 100 trillion), it's probably not surprising that numerous candida symptoms involve the gut. Frequent digestive symptoms related to candida are:

Food Cravings. When candida grows out of control, it continually urges you to give it what it needs and wants: more sugar and refined carbohydrates.

Constipation. A normal, healthy gut will produce one or two bowel movements per day. Dysbiosis and leaky gut caused by candida can lead to constipation—infrequent bowel movements—which can be very uncomfortable.

Diarrhea. Constipation and diarrhea are two sides of the same coin. In some cases, intestinal dysbiosis may cause diarrhea. Diarrhea often occurs when the body is trying to rid itself of an infection or allergen and, in the case of candida, it can be your body's way of attempting to eliminate the candida organisms.

Bloating and Gas. When food isn't digested properly or ferments in the digestive tract, bloating and gas emissions can occur.

Cramps. Abdominal pain, which can occur anywhere along the digestive tract, can be a sign that candida has taken over the intestines.

When Should I See a Doctor?

Although many candida patients can effectively treat their symptoms through dietary changes, I encourage everyone to visit their medical doctor for advice before beginning any new treatment or diet. If you suspect you have an acute candida infection, such as a yeast infection or oral thrush, visit your doctor if you:

- Experience strange or bloody vaginal discharge
- Experience frequent urination
- Have pain in the genitals
- See white sores in your mouth, along with redness and pain
- Experience fever or chills

In some cases, even when employing your best dietary and lifestyle efforts, a medical drug might be necessary. The type of medication and dosage will depend on your unique situation. Some of the medications available include: antifungal drugs such as azoles and echinocandins, which prevent candida organisms from building their cell membranes and low-strength corticosteroids, which reduce the inflammation and itching that comes along with candida infections. Some of these are available over the counter, while others require a doctor's prescription, so speak to your health-care practitioner about your options.

If you are also working with a naturopath or another alternative health practitioner, they might recommend antifungal herbs to inhibit further candida growth. You should work with a health practitioner to make sure you are taking the right herbs in the right amount so they don't negatively affect your medical treatment.

Using Food to Address the Symptoms of Candida

Diet plays an important role in the development and management of candida. Although a candida-free diet may seem restrictive at first, it's important to remember that you can eat a wide array of delicious food. Besides, good health is a far more satisfying reward than a candy bar, don't you think?

Eating to Starve Candida

Our bodies contain a wide variety of bacteria, which play myriad roles in the body. They enhance immune function, boost the absorption and assimilation of nutrients, produce vitamins (particularly B vitamins and vitamin K), break down and build hormones, regulate bowel movements, and keep bad bacteria in check.

Yeast overgrowth occurs when there is an imbalance of bacteria in the gut. Ideally, we want a ratio of roughly 80 percent good bacteria to 20 percent bad bacteria. When an event, or series of events, tips the balance of intestinal flora, a multitude of health issues can arise. The instigator of this imbalance might be a consistently poor diet, a round of antibiotics, a period of extreme stress, or a preexisting health condition that leaves you vulnerable, like diabetes or an autoimmune condition.

The foods we eat play a large role in maintaining and building our intestinal health, which can prevent candida from occurring in the first place or can assist with intestinal healing and eliminating candida overgrowth. If our diet lacks fresh vegetables, good sources of fat and protein, immune-supportive foods, liver-supportive foods, antifungal foods, and fermented foods (which are natural probiotic sources), we leave ourselves vulnerable to an imbalance of beneficial bacteria in the gut. If there is a decrease in the good gut bacteria, candida can pounce, take control, and grow wildly. However, when we starve the body of the foods that candida loves (the sugary, starchy foods), it begins to die, priming the good bacteria to take over once again.

Foods to Avoid

There are many foods that can stimulate candida growth, such as the ones listed below:

- Agave
- Alcohol
- Bread
- Caffeine
- Cakes
- Cashews
- Chocolate and candy
- Cookies
- Dairy products (all)

- Dates
- Dried fruits
- Fermented foods, such as sauerkraut, yogurt, kefir, kombucha, pickles
- Flours/refined flours
- Fruit (all) *except* lemon and lime
- Gluten/glutenous grains
- Honey
- Miso
- Mushrooms
- Pasta
- Peanuts
- Pistachios
- Soy sauce/tamari
- Sucanat
- Sugar: coconut, date, white
- Syrup: coconut, corn, maple
- Vinegar
- Yeast

Foods to Enjoy

I recommend that people buy as much organic food as they can afford, but I realize this is not within everyone's budget. A top priority when seeking out organic or wild items should be given to animal products and fish. Factory-farmed meat and fish products are often loaded with preservatives, hormones, antibiotics, and grains. For produce, I recommend choosing fresh or frozen.

- Almonds
- Amaranth
- Artichokes
- Asparagus
- Avocado
- Beef
- Bone broth
- Brown rice
- Buckwheat
- Chicken
- Coconut products (meat, oil)
- Dark leafy greens (all)
- Eggplant
- Eggs
- Fennel
- Fish
- Garlic
- Herbs and spices, especially basil, cinnamon, cloves, dill, ginger, oregano, rosemary, sage, thyme
- Lamb
- Oats, gluten-free
- Oil: camelina (an oil rich in omega-3 fatty acids from the camelina plant), flax, hemp, olive
- Olives
- Onions
- Pecans
- Quinoa
- Seaweed
- Seeds: chia, hemp, pumpkin (shelled), sunflower (shelled)
- Squashes
- Stevia
- Teff (a gluten-free grain)
- Tomatoes
- Turkey
- Vegetables, cruciferous (all)
- Vegetables, root, starchy (roots and squash in moderation)
- Walnuts

Harnessing the Power of Probiotics

Probiotics are friendly bacteria that aid digestion, support the immune system, help manufacture vitamins, and police the unhealthy bacteria to keep them from growing. Once the candida organisms have diminished, it's important to repopulate and nourish the digestive tract with beneficial flora that work to prevent candida from conquering the gut in the future.

Probiotics, even if you are taking antibiotics or antifungals, can help repopulate the digestive tract with good bacteria and prevent further overgrowth. In studies where probiotics and antibiotics were administered together, researchers showed that probiotics are still effective when used in conjunction with antibiotics and can even reduce an antibiotic's side effects, enhance its function, and improve immunity.

If you are not taking an antibiotic, I don't see any reason not to include a good probiotic as part of your candida protocol. Probiotic supplements are a great addition throughout the three phases outlined on page 12 and support to the recipes in this book.

You can take probiotics in two ways: in supplements and in fermented foods. There are so many probiotic supplements on store shelves, making a choice can be confusing. Two types of probiotics, *lactobacillus acidophilus* and *Bifidobacterium bifidum*, are especially helpful in addressing candida and promoting a healthy intestinal environment. Recommended dosages vary—I recommend working with a health practitioner to determine the dose that's right for you. Make sure to store your supplements properly to maintain their effectiveness and shelf life.

You can also find probiotics in naturally fermented foods, such as:

- Cultured (or fermented) vegetables
- Kimchi
- Kombucha
- Miso
- Sauerkraut
- Tempeh
- Dairy-Free Yogurt

I offer a few caveats for using fermented foods with candida. If you're not used to consuming fermented foods, the high amount of probiotics in them can cause gastrointestinal upset. Fermented foods purchased at the grocery store can also be loaded with sugar, particularly foods like yogurt, kombucha, or cultured vegetables. And since sugar feeds candida, we don't want to consume those sugary fermented foods.

That's why I recommend leaving out fermented foods in the detox phase, Phase 1: Repair, of a candida-free diet. Then I add them later—preferably homemade versions to eliminate unwanted ingredients. Chapter 9, Fermented Foods, offers some easy and delicious recipes to help you do just that.

The Three Phases of a Candida-Free Diet

Now it's time to put our knowledge to work in creating an action plan that will reduce candida, support your health, and allow you to eat delicious foods while doing so. This chapter details the three-phase process you can apply to start beating candida—Phase 1: Repair; Phase 2: Rebuild; and Phase 3: Revitalize—along with foods to include in each step. By removing certain foods, you can starve the candida in your body of its food source, and then rebuild gut health by continuing to avoid certain foods while adding others to the diet.

I strongly recommend sticking to Phase 1 for a minimum of one month. Phase 2: Rebuild is generally two weeks. If you move from one phase to the next and immediately notice that your symptoms reemerge, that is a sign you are not ready for new foods, so you should return to the previous phase.

You are your own best health practitioner, so do what feels right for you.

Phase 1: Repair

In Phase 1, we aim to starve the candida of its main fuel source: sugars and starches. Most of this phase involves consuming fresh vegetables, nuts, seeds, fish, sea vegetables, and meat (see Foods to Enjoy on page 10).

There are beneficial aspects to produce like root vegetables and gluten-free whole grains, so I recommend consuming sweeter vegetables such as carrots, yams, parsnips, and beets in moderation during the first phase of the diet, keeping to about *½ cup per day*, total. If you don't have a problem complying to addition dietary restrictions, go ahead and eliminate these foods. During Phase 1, I also recommend taking a daily probiotic to encourage the growth of beneficial bacteria in the digestive tract.

Phase 1 of the diet is the most difficult, particularly if you have been eating a lot of starchy carbohydrates or if you are not used to healthy eating or cooking. You may experience gastrointestinal upset, aches and pains, headaches, mood swings, skin rashes, fatigue, or food cravings as your body begins to rid itself of candida. It's likely you'll feel worse before you start to feel better. This is to be expected, so don't worry. Everyone has different symptoms, and the severity varies as well. Here are some ways to deal with some of the challenges of Phase 1:

Replace snacking with another ritual. If you have a habit of eating treats on a break, do something else instead: have a cup of tea, go for a walk, or call a friend.

Try gentle exercise. Gentle exercise such as walking or yoga can help get your blood flowing, encourage the release of toxins, and help calm you.

Take deep breaths. Breathing and meditation helps oxygenate your tissues and reduce stress.

Drink plenty of water. Water helps you feel full, plus it encourages elimination and sweeps the toxins out.

Phase 2: Rebuild

Phase 2 of the diet is similar to Phase 1. We continue to avoid foods that encourage candida growth, and we add some fermented and low-glycemic foods.

Once there has been a significant amount of candida die-off, it's important to begin rebuilding the community of beneficial organisms in your gut. Although fermented foods are too unpredictable to include in Phase 1, we can now begin to include them in the diet. Following are the foods we can begin to add to menu plans:

- Low-glycemic fruits: berries (blackberry, blueberry, cranberry, raspberry, strawberry), green apple, pear, cherries, plums
- Beans/legumes (black beans, kidney beans, lentils, lima beans, navy beans)
- Raw, homemade nondairy yogurt (avoid sugary brands at the grocery store; see page 120 to learn how to make yogurt at home)
- Raw apple cider vinegar: this boosts stomach acid, contains friendly bacteria, and helps balance blood sugar
- Small portions of fermented foods (kimchi, kombucha, miso, pickles, sauerkraut, tempeh, yogurt; avoid sugar brands at the grocery store and make sure to pick brands fermented in salt, not vinegar)
- Maintain supplementation with probiotics

In Phase 2, I hope you're feeling pretty good—with regular bowel movements, more energy, fewer aches and pains. All your symptoms might not be 100 percent gone, or some days you might feel fantastic while others are more of a challenge. That's okay. The goal is to keep fostering health and wellness, and each bite of healthy food you take will help you do this.

I encourage you to experiment with the foods we add into Phase 2 and see whether they work for you. You won't know if a food is helpful to you until you try it, so start sampling. Add foods one at a time, and then wait three days so you can discern which foods might be a problem.

Phase 3: Revitalize

By the third phase, I expect that your candida symptoms are under control and you feel confident exploring a wider range of foods. Congratulations!

Phase 3: Revitalize invites you to maintain your diet and prepare for anti-candida eating for the long haul. Remember, if you return to your old ways of consuming refined sugary treats, you will create an internal environment that may encourage candida to return. That means there are certain foods you should continue to avoid, such as candy, white sugar, refined foods, processed foods, and gluten, as well as starchy carbohydrates like white rice, potatoes, and white bread. I also recommend avoiding conventional dairy products, since they are packed with sugars and are challenging to digest.

In Phase 3, begin adding the following items to your meals:

- Small portions of sweeter fruits—small portions, ½ cup serving per day (like bananas, kiwi, mango, nectarines, papaya, peaches, pineapple)
- Whole-grain gluten-free flours (such as amaranth, brown rice, buckwheat, chickpea, millet, sorghum)
- Whole-food sweeteners, like dates and raw honey (experiment with small amounts)
- Dried fruit
- Try adding foods with yeast, mushrooms, vinegars, cashews, and pistachios, if you are symptom free for at least six months
- Sweeter vegetables, such as root vegetables and squash (remove the limits)
- Fermented foods and daily probiotic supplementation (continue with)

Be alert for any symptoms that emerge as you test new foods. Following any type of elimination diet often cleanses the body and leaves you with a fresh slate—even if you've had that food in the past, you may not be able to tolerate it any longer. Continue maintaining a healthy diet to prevent candida from taking over in the future. Remember, our guts are inextricably linked to overall good health, so continue to consume food and drinks that help your body.

Frequently Asked Questions about Candida

Can pregnant women follow the candida-free diet?

I would not recommend that pregnant women follow the candida-free diet as outlined in this book. When on the diet, our bodies begin to detoxify, and that process will release toxins into the body. With pregnant women, I would be concerned about the effect of these toxins on the fetus. However, pregnant women can abide by a modified version of the diet—for example, cutting out refined sugars, processed foods, baked treats, yeast, caffeine, and white potatoes. Focusing on low-glycemic fruits is also an option, instead of removing the fruit category completely.

How long will it take for my symptoms to go away?

After the initial candida die-off phase, which lasts about a couple of weeks, hopefully you will begin to see results within a month. Your health issues won't all magically disappear—building health takes time and effort—but you should see an improvement and continue to improve as you follow the diet. The stricter you are with the diet, the quicker you'll see results.

I'm vegan. Can I still follow a candida-free diet?

Yes. It can be more challenging to follow a candida-free diet as a vegan. Some foods that vegans tend to eat in large quantities—grains, pasta, breads, beans, and legumes—can be processed and starchy and are not recommended in the initial stage of the diet. Vegans need to be more mindful of consuming enough nutrients, so in the first phase of the diet, you will be focusing on eating fresh vegetables; non-moldy nuts; high-protein seeds like hemp, chia, and flax; good sources of fat; and nutrient-rich seaweed. Then, in later stages, vegans can add in fruit and legumes.

Cooking in the Candida-Free Kitchen

Many packaged and takeout foods contain ingredients that feed candida, so a candida-free diet involves plenty of home cooking. To set yourself up for success, equip yourself with the kitchen essentials that will make cooking easier.

Equipment Essentials

A blender. A good blender helps make delicious soups, smoothies, juices, dips, nut and seed milks, puddings, ice cream, and more.

A good knife. Healthy cooking inevitably involves plenty of slicing, dicing, and chopping. Find a good, all-purpose chef's knife that will help you cut a variety of vegetables, herbs, and meats.

Food processor. Food processors are great for making foods that are thicker in texture such as homemade nut and seed butters, blitzing burger patties (both veggie and meat), and pulsing mixtures for raw, rolled snack bars.

Pots and pans. You don't need a fancy eighteen-piece set of matching cookware, but I recommend purchasing a small pot, a medium pot, a large pot, and a large frying or sauté pan. These equip you with what you need to prepare a wide variety of meals. I recommend using stainless steel, ceramic, or cast-iron pots and pans.

Rimmed baking sheets. These are perfect for roasting vegetables; toasting nuts, grains, and spices; making baked goods, oven fries, and granola; broiling fish and meat; and reheating foods. If I'm making something I don't want to stick to the pan, I'll use a silicone baking mat, aluminum foil, or unbleached parchment paper for easy cleanup.

Refrigerator Essentials

- Almond milk and unsweetened coconut milk
- Eggs
- Fish (like halibut or salmon)
- Fresh herbs (like basil, cilantro, and thyme)
- Fruits (like lemons, limes, and tomatoes)
- Meat (like beef, chicken, lamb, and turkey)
- Veggies (like asparagus, bell peppers, carrots, celery, eggplant, garlic, kale, onions, and spinach)

Pantry Essentials

- Almond flour and coconut flour
- Apple cider vinegar (not for Phase 1)
- Broth
- Brown rice and quinoa
- Coconut oil and olive oil
- Legumes (like chickpeas or navy beans; not for Phase 1)
- Nuts and seeds (like almonds, walnuts, sesame seeds, and sunflower seeds; avoid peanuts)
- Oats
- Spices and dried herbs (like cinnamon, cloves, dill, ginger, oregano, pepper, rosemary, sage, and salt)
- Stevia
- Vanilla extract

The Recipes in This Book

Now that you know the details of the candida-free diet, it is time to delve into the fun part of any culinary journey—the recipes. These recipes are labeled as Phase 1, with tips on how to create a Phase 2 dish, and Phase 3 recipes. Always use the freshest ingredients possible. When you have to purchase processed ingredients, such as chicken or beef broth, look at the nutrition data carefully to ensure the product is *gluten-free and additive-free, as well as organic*. Don't be afraid to substitute ingredients in a recipe for family favorites or what you have available. Cooking is supposed to be an enjoyable and creative process.

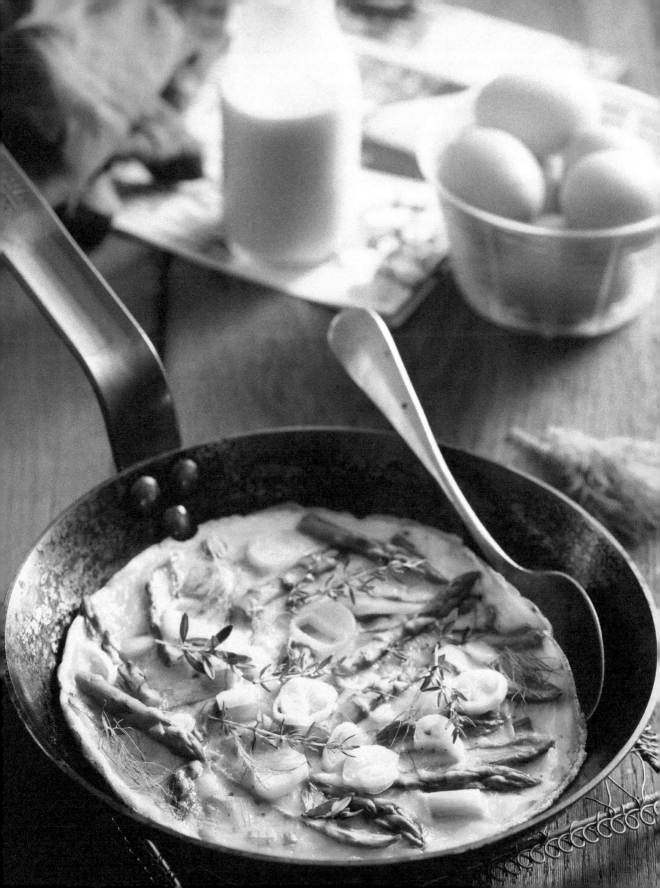

Chapter 2

Breakfast and Smoothies

Cool Cucumber-Herb Smoothie

SERVES 2 / PREP: 5 MINUTES

Smoothies are often more like a dessert than a main meal because of the copious bananas and tablespoons of honey some people put in to disguise the flavor of greens like kale and spinach. You might be surprised how little you miss the sugary taste when enjoying fresh cucumber and herbs instead. The listed herbs can be swapped out for others, such as dill, savory, marjoram, and chives.

1 English cucumber, chopped

1 cup shredded kale

½ cup coconut water

1 teaspoon chopped fresh basil

1 teaspoon chopped fresh thyme

½ teaspoon chopped fresh oregano

Pinch sea salt

4 ice cubes

1. In a blender, purée the cucumber, kale, coconut water, basil, thyme, oregano, and sea salt until blended.

2. Add the ice and blend until thick and smooth.

3. Serve.

PHASE 1: (Per Serving) Calories: 57; Total Fat: 0g; Saturated Fat: 0g; Carbohydrates: 13g; Fiber: 2g; Protein: 2g

PHASE 2: (Per Serving) Calories: 57; Total Fat: 0g; Saturated Fat: 0g; Carbohydrates: 13g; Fiber: 2g; Protein: 2g

PHASE 2 TIP: Add 1 teaspoon of raw apple cider vinegar to complement the crisp flavor of the cucumber.

Sunny Butternut Squash Smoothie

SERVES 2 / PREP: 5 MINUTES

Lots of leftover squash can be the result when you roast or purée it for supper, because these beautifully colored vegetables can be very large. Blending leftovers for breakfast with protein-packed pumpkin seeds and warm spices is a perfect solution. You might find yourself hunting through the produce section for a huge squash just to create leftovers because this smoothie is so delicious and satisfying.

2 cups cooked, mashed butternut squash

1 cup unsweetened coconut milk

2 tablespoons shelled pumpkin seeds (pepitas)

1 (7-g) packet stevia

½ teaspoon ground nutmeg

¼ teaspoon ground cinnamon

Pinch ground allspice

4 ice cubes

1. In a blender, purée the squash, coconut milk, pumpkin seeds, stevia, nutmeg, cinnamon, and allspice until smooth.

2. Add the ice and purée until thick and blended. Serve.

PHASE 1: (Per Serving) Calories: 310; Total Fat: 13g; Saturated Fat: 6g; Carbohydrates: 51g; Fiber: 16g; Protein: 8g

PHASE 2: (Per Serving) Calories: 358; Total Fat: 13g; Saturated Fat: 6g; Carbohydrates: 64g; Fiber: 18g; Protein: 8g

PHASE 2 TIP: Add ½ of a peeled green apple for extra fiber and nutrients.

Chia Power Smoothie

SERVES 1 / PREP: 5 MINUTES

Chia seeds are often used in recipes for their thickening power; they form a thick gel when soaked in liquid. So, if you want a thicker smoothie, you can use two methods to get stellar results. You can blend all the ingredients except the ice and let the smoothie sit for 30 minutes before blending in the ice, or you can add the chia seeds to the coconut water and let that mixture sit for 30 minutes before blending all the ingredients together.

1 cup coconut water

2 celery stalks

1 cup shredded spinach

½ English cucumber

2 tablespoons chia seeds

1 tablespoon freshly squeezed lime juice

1 tablespoon chopped fresh basil

Pinch sea salt

3 ice cubes

1. In a blender, purée the coconut water, celery, spinach, cucumber, chia seeds, lime juice, basil, and sea salt.

2. Add the ice cubes and purée until thick and smooth. Serve.

PHASE 1: (Per Serving) Calories: 165; Total Fat: 5g; Saturated Fat: 0g; Carbohydrates: 32g; Fiber: 7g; Protein: 5g

PHASE 2: (Per Serving) Calories: 188; Total Fat: 6g; Saturated Fat: 0g; Carbohydrates: 38g; Fiber: 9g; Protein: 6g

PHASE 2 TIP: Add ½ cup of fresh or frozen strawberries.

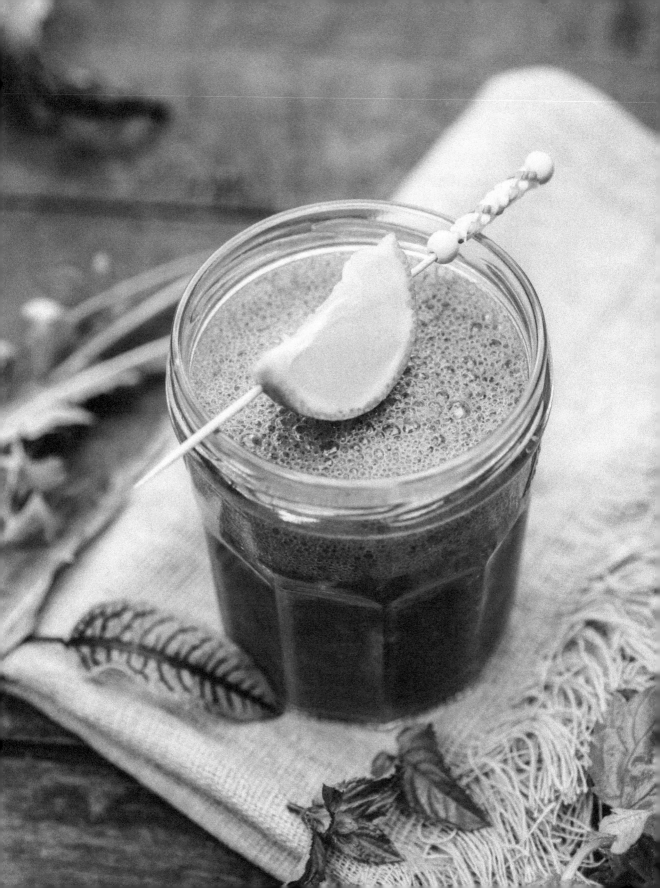

Bircher Muesli

SERVES 4 / PREP: 10 MINUTES + OVERNIGHT SOAKING TIME

When staying in Europe, especially in Germanic countries, you will find this nutty, creamy dish on the menu everywhere. It is like a cold porridge with lots of texture and many flavors. The dry ingredients can be doubled or tripled and stored in a sealed container for up to one month if you want a quick and healthy meal choice. Simply measure the quantity you want and add homemade yogurt, unsweetened almond milk, or unsweetened coconut milk until you have the desired consistency.

1 cup unsweetened shredded coconut

½ cup slivered almonds

½ cup chopped walnuts

¼ cup gluten-free rolled oats

¼ cup chia seeds

½ teaspoon ground cinnamon

¼ teaspoon ground nutmeg

Pinch sea salt

1½ cups Homemade Coconut Yogurt (page 120)

1 cup unsweetened almond milk

1. In a large bowl, stir together the coconut, almonds, walnuts, oats, chia seeds, cinnamon, nutmeg, and sea salt until well mixed.

2. Stir in the yogurt and almond milk.

3. Cover the bowl and refrigerate overnight to soften. Serve.

(Per Serving) Calories: 515; Total Fat: 42g; Saturated Fat: 20g; Carbohydrates: 26g; Fiber: 10g; Protein: 13g

INGREDIENT TIP: Take care when purchasing oats. Although oats are naturally gluten-free, they are often packaged in manufacturing plants that also handle wheat products. Look for a label that indicates the produce was packaged in a gluten-free facility and do not buy oats in a bulk store where cross contamination is common.

Oatmeal Breakfast Pudding

SERVES 2 / PREP: 15 MINUTES + 1 HOUR CHILLING TIME

This is more like a chia pudding than oatmeal, but the oats do add a familiar texture and look to the dish. If you want an exceptional taste, place a large dry skillet over low heat and lightly toast the oats by swirling the pan until they are golden and fragrant. If you are in Phase 3 of the candida-free diet, a little raw honey or chopped dates instead of stevia is a lovely addition.

1½ cups unsweetened coconut milk

½ cup chia seeds

½ cup gluten-free rolled oats

¼ cup shelled unsalted sunflower seeds

2 teaspoons granulated stevia

1 teaspoon alcohol-free vanilla extract

½ teaspoon ground cinnamon

⅛ teaspoon ground cloves

1. In a medium bowl, stir together the coconut milk, chia seeds, oats, sunflower seeds, stevia, vanilla, cinnamon, and cloves until very well mixed.

2. Refrigerate for at least 1 hour so the chia seeds soak up the coconut milk. Serve.

PHASE 1: (Per Serving) Calories: 281; Total Fat: 18g; Saturated Fat: 4g; Carbohydrates: 31g; Fiber: 14g; Protein: 11g

PHASE 2: (Per Serving) Calories: 304; Total Fat: 18g; Saturated Fat: 4g; Carbohydrates: 38g; Fiber: 15g; Protein: 11g

PHASE 2 TIP: Add ½ of a green apple, shredded, to the mixture with ¼ teaspoon of freshly squeezed lemon juice before placing the bowl in the refrigerator to soak.

Multigrain Porridge

SERVES 4 / PREP: 5 MINUTES / COOK: 15 MINUTES

Many people associate porridge with instant packaged cereal that requires water and turns out gluey and tooth-achingly sweet. Porridge should be wholesome, provide lots of energy without spiking blood sugar, and take more time than a couple of minutes in the microwave to cook. The buckwheat groats in this version add an interesting, complex flavor and lots of fiber and minerals to start your day. Buckwheat is also gluten-free.

½ cup gluten-free rolled oats

½ cup shelled pumpkin seeds (pepitas)

½ cup buckwheat groats

¼ cup chopped pecans

¼ cup dried cranberries

2 teaspoons granulated stevia

½ teaspoon ground cinnamon

¼ teaspoon ground cardamom

¼ teaspoon ground ginger

Pinch ground cloves

3 cups unsweetened almond milk

1 teaspoon alcohol-free vanilla extract

1. In a large saucepan, stir together the oats, pumpkin seeds, buckwheat, pecans, cranberries, stevia, cinnamon, cardamom, ginger, and cloves.

2. Add the almond milk and vanilla. Stir until the mixture is blended.

3. Place the saucepan over medium heat. Bring the porridge to a simmer, stirring constantly, and then reduce the heat to low and simmer for about 15 minutes, or until it is the desired consistency.

4. Remove from the heat and serve.

(Per Serving) Calories: 267; Total Fat: 14g; Saturated Fat: 2g; Carbohydrates: 29g; Fiber: 6g; Protein: 10g

Buckwheat Pancakes

SERVES 4 / PREP: 10 MINUTES / COOK: 20 MINUTES

Lazy Sunday mornings seem like the best time to mix up the batter for golden pancakes to serve to family or special guests. Buckwheat is a popular choice for pancake enthusiasts because this fruit seed has an assertive, almost toasty flavor that is accented beautifully by yogurt and a touch of raw honey, and is gluten-free. Sliced peaches or pitted black cherries are wonderful toppings, in addition to the berries.

1 cup buckwheat flour

½ teaspoon baking powder

½ teaspoon baking soda

Pinch sea salt

1¼ cups unsweetened almond milk

¼ cup Homemade Coconut Yogurt (page 120)

1 large egg

1 tablespoon raw honey

Coconut oil, for the pan

2 cups mixed berries

1. In a small bowl, stir together the buckwheat flour, baking powder, baking soda, and sea salt.

2. In a large bowl, whisk together the almond milk, yogurt, egg, and honey until well blended.

3. Whisk the buckwheat mixture into the milk mixture until smooth.

4. Place a large skillet over medium heat and lightly brush it with coconut oil.

5. Pour out 4 pancakes into the skillet using ¼ cup of batter for each. Cook the pancakes for about 3 minutes, or until the edges are firm and the bottom is golden. Flip the pancakes over and cook for about 2 minutes more, or until the other side is golden.

6. Remove the pancakes to a warm plate and repeat with the remaining batter.

7. Serve 3 pancakes per person, topped with ½ cup of berries.

(Per Serving) Calories: 213; Total Fat: 6g; Saturated Fat: 2g; Carbohydrates: 37g; Fiber: 5g; Protein: 7g

Baked French Toast

SERVES 2 / PREP: 15 MINUTES + 10 MINUTES SOAKING TIME / COOK: 30 MINUTES

If you need more portions of this simple dish, double the recipe and layer the extra bread on top of the first set. You are basically making a bread pudding without cutting up the bread. You can also assemble the entire recipe the evening before and pop it in the oven in the morning straight from the refrigerator. Try substituting unsweetened coconut milk for the almond milk and topping the French toast with a sprinkle of shredded unsweetened coconut.

Coconut oil, for the baking dish

4 gluten-free bread slices

2 large eggs

½ cup unsweetened almond milk

2 teaspoons granulated stevia

1 teaspoon alcohol-free vanilla extract

½ teaspoon ground cinnamon

¼ teaspoon ground nutmeg

1. Preheat the oven to 350°F.

2. Coat an 8-by-8-inch baking dish with coconut oil.

3. In the prepared dish, arrange the bread slices in a single layer with a little overlap, if necessary.

4. In a medium bowl, whisk together the eggs, almond milk, stevia, vanilla, cinnamon, and nutmeg until well mixed.

5. Pour the egg mixture evenly over the bread. Let it sit for 10 minutes to soak into the bread.

6. Place in the preheated oven and bake for about 30 minutes, or until the bread is golden. Serve warm.

(Per Serving) Calories: 248; Total Fat: 11g; Saturated Fat: 2g; Carbohydrates: 28g; Fiber: 4g; Protein: 7g

Summer Herb Omelet

SERVES 3 / PREP: 15 MINUTES / COOK: 10 MINUTES

Egg white omelets were all the rage in the 1980s and 1990s when fat was the enemy and egg yolks equaled skyrocketing cholesterol in the public's mind. Eggs have made a comeback as a healthy choice since recent scientific research has established their healthy attributes. This is not solely an egg white omelet, since there is one whole egg in the mix, but the snowy-white color looks gorgeous, and tastes great, paired on the plate with the fragrant green herbs.

9 large egg whites

1 large egg

1 tablespoon chopped fresh parsley

1 teaspoon chopped fresh thyme

1 teaspoon chopped fresh basil

1 tablespoon olive oil

1 scallion, chopped

Sea salt

Freshly ground black pepper

1. In a large bowl, whisk together the egg whites, egg, parsley, thyme, and basil until well blended. Set aside.

2. Place a large skillet over medium heat and add the olive oil.

3. Add the scallion, and sauté for about 2 minutes, or until softened.

4. Pour the egg mixture into the skillet and cook, swirling the skillet, for about 3 minutes, or until the edges start to set. Lift the set edges with a spatula and tilt the pan so the uncooked egg flows under the cooked egg. Continue swirling, lifting, and cooking the egg until the omelet is just set, about 4 minutes.

5. Loosen the omelet with a spatula and fold it in half. Cut the folded omelet into 3 portions and transfer to serving plates. Season with sea salt and pepper and serve.

(Per Serving) Calories: 118; Total Fat: 7g; Saturated Fat: 1g; Carbohydrates: 1g; Fiber: 0g; Protein: 13g

Baked Egg Skillet

SERVES 4 / PREP: 10 MINUTES / COOK: 26 MINUTES

Antique stores and interesting eclectic secondhand stores are perfect locations to unearth authentic cast-iron skillets for all your cooking needs, like this colorful breakfast dish. Cast iron can certainly be found in modern stores, but scrubbing, seasoning, and polishing an old relic can be very satisfying. If you do not have a cast-iron skillet, you can certainly use a more contemporary pan with nice results.

1 tablespoon olive oil

1 leek, white and light green parts, sliced thin

2 cups asparagus spears, cut into 1-inch pieces

½ sweet onion, chopped

½ teaspoon minced garlic

6 large eggs, beaten

½ cup unsweetened almond milk

½ teaspoon chopped fresh dill

½ teaspoon chopped fresh thyme

Pinch sea salt

Pinch freshly ground black pepper

Dill or thyme sprigs, for garnish

1. Preheat the oven to 375°F.

2. Place a large ovenproof skillet over medium heat and add the olive oil. Add the leek, asparagus, onion, and garlic and sauté for about 6 minutes, or until softened.

3. In a medium bowl, whisk together the beaten eggs, almond milk, dill, thyme, sea salt, and pepper.

4. Pour the eggs into the skillet, shaking it to distribute the liquid among the vegetables. Place in the preheated oven and bake for about 20 minutes, or until the eggs are set and lightly golden.

5. Top with dill or thyme sprigs, or both, and serve.

PHASE 1: (Per Serving) Calories: 187; Total Fat: 12g; Saturated Fat: 3g; Carbohydrates: 10g; Fiber: 3g; Protein: 13g

PHASE 2: (Per Serving) Calories: 243; Total Fat: 12g; Saturated Fat: 3g; Carbohydrates: 20g; Fiber: 7g; Protein: 17g

PHASE 2 TIP: Add 1 cup of cooked red lentils to the vegetables.

Tomato-Pepper Poached Eggs

SERVES 2 / PREP: 10 MINUTES / COOK: 15 MINUTES

Professional chefs practice poaching with countless eggs to get the perfect shape, texture, and a velvety runny yolk. You can create poached eggs that rival a chef's simply by cracking them into this fragrant tomato mixture and popping the whole pan in the oven. The eggs poach evenly in the piping-hot sauce, and you don't have to waste cartons of eggs to get there.

1 tablespoon olive oil

1 small sweet onion, chopped

1 red bell pepper, chopped

1 teaspoon minced garlic

2 large tomatoes, chopped, with juices

1 tablespoon chopped fresh basil

1 teaspoon chopped fresh oregano

Pinch red pepper flakes

Pinch sea salt

Pinch freshly ground black pepper

4 large eggs

1. Place a large lidded skillet over medium heat and add the olive oil. Add the onion, bell pepper, and garlic and sauté for about 4 minutes, or until the vegetables soften.

2. Add the tomatoes and their juices, basil, oregano, red pepper flakes, sea salt, and black pepper. Bring the mixture to a simmer. Reduce the heat to low and simmer for 5 minutes.

3. With the back of a large spoon, make 4 wells in the tomato sauce. Crack 1 egg into each well and place a lid on the skillet.

4. Poach the eggs for about 5 minutes, or until the whites are set and the yolks are still runny. Serve the eggs with the sauce.

PHASE 1: (Per Serving) Calories: 273; Total Fat: 18g; Saturated Fat: 4g; Carbohydrates: 16g; Fiber: 5g; Protein: 15g

PHASE 2: (Per Serving) Calories: 275; Total Fat: 18g; Saturated Fat: 4g; Carbohydrates: 16g; Fiber: 5g; Protein: 15g

PHASE 2 TIP: Add 1 tablespoon of raw apple cider vinegar to the sauce with the tomatoes and herbs. You can serve this delectable dish on gluten-free toast for a more substantial meal.

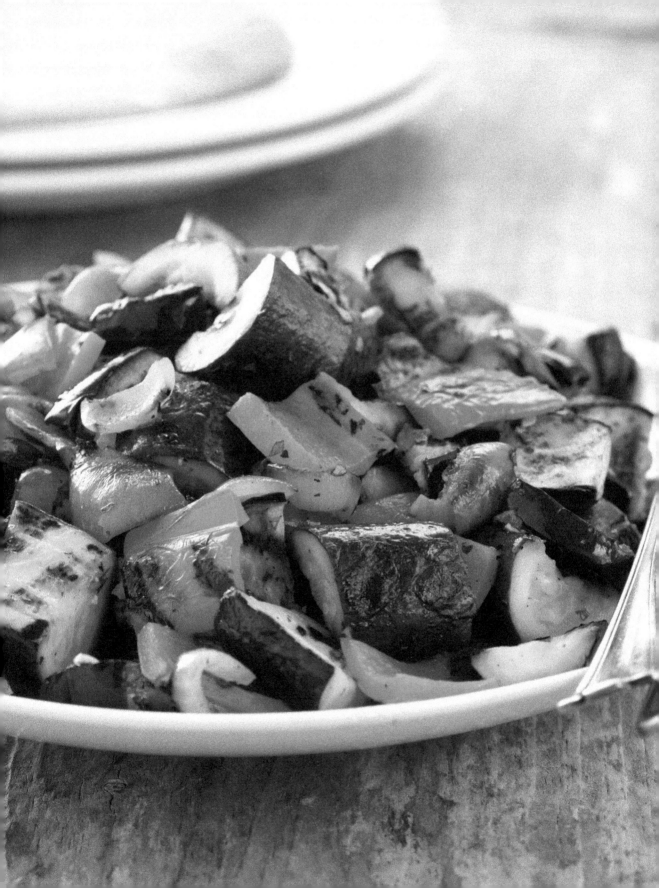

Chapter 3

Snacks and Sides

Open-Faced Egg Bruschetta

SERVES 4 / PREP: 5 MINUTES / COOK: 10 MINUTES

Golden, dripping egg yolks, bright-green vegetables, juicy tomatoes, and crispy toasted bread make a perfect choice for after-school snacks, late-night munchies, or a midmorning bit of energy. If you have the time, and a barbecue, grill the bread instead of toasting it after lightly brushing both sides with olive oil. The rich, charred flavor sets off the other recipe components nicely.

1 tablespoon olive oil, divided

1 cup shredded kale

4 artichoke hearts, chopped

4 large eggs

4 gluten-free bread slices, toasted

8 thin tomato slices, divided

Pinch sea salt

Pinch freshly ground black pepper

1 tablespoon chopped fresh parsley

1. Place a large skillet over medium heat and add 2 teaspoons of olive oil. Add the kale and artichoke hearts and sauté for about 5 minutes, or until tender. Transfer the sautéed vegetables to a bowl and set aside.

2. Wipe out the skillet. Add the remaining 1 teaspoon of olive oil and place the skillet back over medium heat.

3. Crack the eggs into the skillet and fry them, sunny-side up, for about 4 minutes, or until the whites are set and the yolks are still runny.

4. Top each slice of toast with 2 tomato slices. Season with the sea salt and pepper. Add one-quarter of the cooked vegetables to each piece. Top each with 1 cooked egg and garnish with parsley.

(Per Serving) Calories: 269; Total Fat: 11g; Saturated Fat: 2g; Carbohydrates: 33g; Fiber: 11g; Protein: 12g

PHASE 1 **PHASE 2**

Tomato-Scallion Salsa

MAKES 2 CUPS / PREP: 5 MINUTES

Salsa seems like a basic recipe: just cut up a bunch of vegetables and mix them together in a bowl. There is, however, an art to combining textures, sweetness, and a hint of spice or heat to create a satisfying blend. If you enjoy hot peppers, mince your favorite chile and add it with the other ingredients. Leftover salsa can be spooned over baked or grilled fish as a main course.

3 large tomatoes, chopped

½ yellow bell pepper, chopped

½ small English cucumber, chopped

2 scallions, chopped

½ cup chopped fresh cilantro

1 teaspoon minced garlic

½ teaspoon ground cumin

Pinch cayenne pepper

Sea salt, for seasoning

Gluten-free pita bread wedges, for serving

1. In a large bowl, stir together the tomatoes, bell pepper, cucumber, scallions, cilantro, garlic, cumin, and cayenne pepper until mixed.

2. Season with sea salt. Serve with the pita wedges.

PHASE 1: (Per Serving) Calories: 40; Total Fat: 0g; Saturated Fat: 0g; Carbohydrates: 9g; Fiber: 3g; Protein: 2g

PHASE 2: (Per Serving) Calories: 95; Total Fat: 1g; Saturated Fat: 0g; Carbohydrates: 18g; Fiber: 5g; Protein: 5g

PHASE 2 TIP: Add 1 cup of cooked black beans to the salsa.

Chicken Salad Avocado Boats

SERVES 2 / PREP: 5 MINUTES

Avocados make fabulous handy and healthy containers for the other ingredients in this recipe. The fat content of this pale-green fruit helps the body absorb the carotenoids in the kale and red bell pepper along with fat-soluble vitamins such as A and E. The fat in avocados is mostly heart-healthy monounsaturated fat, about 68 percent of the total fat. So, including avocado in your diet can help boost your good (LDL) cholesterol. Avocados also help decrease inflammation in the body and fight antioxidants.

1 cup cooked chopped chicken breast

½ cup chopped red bell pepper

½ cup shredded kale

1 scallion, finely chopped

1 tablespoon chopped fresh cilantro

1 teaspoon freshly squeezed lemon juice

Pinch sea salt

Freshly ground black pepper

1 avocado, peeled, halved, and pitted

1. In a large bowl, stir together the chicken, bell pepper, kale, scallion, cilantro, lemon juice, and sea salt. Season with pepper.

2. Spoon half of the chicken salad into each avocado half and serve.

(PER SERVING) CALORIES: 387; TOTAL FAT: 24G; SATURATED FAT: 5G; CARBOHYDRATES: 15G; FIBER: 8G; PROTEIN: 30G

NUTRITION TIP: When peeling avocados, take care not to remove the dark-green layer of flesh right next to the peel. The majority of the phytonutrients found in avocado are in this area, although the paler flesh closer to the pit is healthy, as well.

Coconut-Ginger Cookies

MAKES 12 COOKIES / PREP: 10 MINUTES / COOK: 10 MINUTES + 15 MINUTES COOLING TIME

If meringues are one of your favorite cookies, you should enjoy this spiked variation that lends to a tender, light cookie. Look for ginger with no greenish areas, no wet or dry spots, and a plump, evenly colored rhizome.

3 large egg whites, at room temperature

Pinch sea salt

1 teaspoon granulated stevia

1 teaspoon alcohol-free vanilla extract

1 teaspoon grated peeled ginger

1½ cups unsweetened shredded coconut

½ cup almond flour

1. Preheat the oven to 350°F. Line a baking sheet with parchment paper and set aside.

2. In a large bowl, beat the egg whites and sea salt with an electric beater until soft peaks form.

3. Beat in the stevia, vanilla, and ginger. Gently fold in the coconut and the almond flour, just until blended.

4. Drop the cookies by tablespoons onto the prepared baking sheet. Place in the preheated oven and bake for about 10 minutes, or until the cookies are light brown.

5. Cool the cookies on the baking sheet for 15 minutes and then transfer to a wire rack to cool completely.

6. Store the cookies in a sealed container at room temperature for up to 4 days.

(Per Serving) Calories: 126; Total Fat: 11g; Saturated Fat: 7g; Carbohydrates: 4g; Fiber: 3g; Protein: 2g

Spicy Bean Dip

SERVES 4 / PREP: 5 MINUTES

Dips seem decadent because they are packed with complex flavors, but this satisfying snack takes very little time to prepare. Navy beans have a mellow taste and creamy, almost buttery, texture when puréed, so this legume makes an ideal base for a dip. The tahini and spices shine through, accented by the fresh tang of lime juice.

2 cups cooked
    navy beans

1 cup cooked chickpeas

1 scallion, chopped

¼ cup tahini
    (sesame paste)

2 tablespoons
    Homemade Coconut
    Yogurt (page 120)

1 tablespoon chopped
    fresh cilantro

2 teaspoons freshly
    squeezed lime juice

1 teaspoon minced garlic

½ teaspoon ground cumin

¼ teaspoon ground
    coriander

Pinch red pepper flakes

Gluten-free pita bread
    wedges, for serving

1. In a food processor, combine the navy beans, chickpeas, scallion, tahini, yogurt, cilantro, lime juice, garlic, cumin, coriander, and red pepper flakes. Pulse until combined but not completely smooth.

2. Transfer the dip to a bowl and serve with the pita wedges.

(Per Serving) Calories: 316; Total Fat: 12g; Saturated Fat: 2g; Carbohydrates: 40g; Fiber: 14g; Protein: 15g

INGREDIENT TIP: Tahini is similar to peanut butter but is made with sesame seeds instead. Purchase tahini that is produced using roasted sesame seeds for a more intense taste.

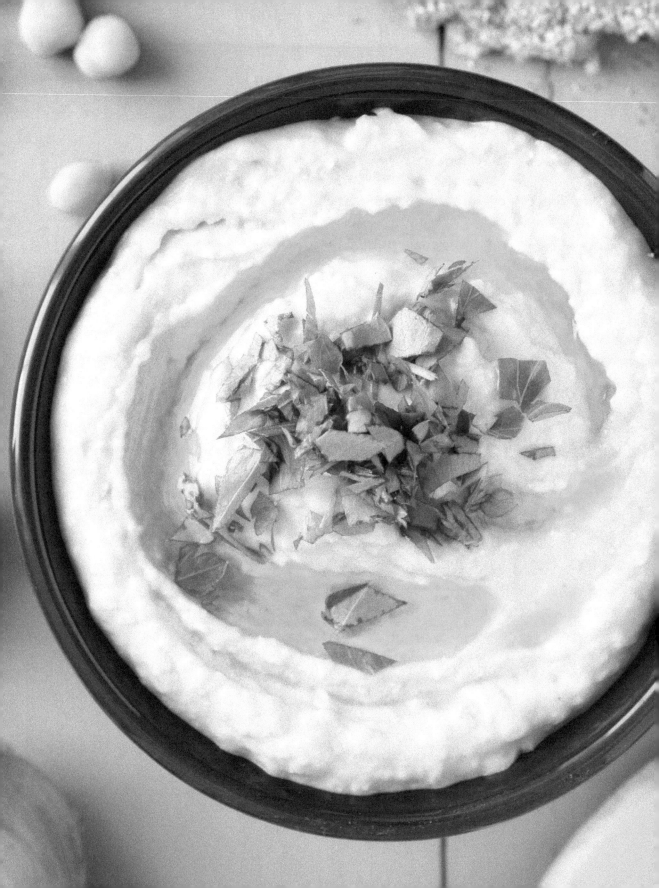

Cumin-Roasted Chickpeas

MAKES 2 CUPS / PREP: 10 MINUTES / COOK: 30 MINUTES

Greasy potato chips, empty-calorie cheese puffs, and additive-coated corn chips are popular snacks because they satisfy cravings for salty, savory foods. Roasted chickpeas can easily take the place of these unhealthy options because their crunch and spicy flavor is perfectly balanced. You can change the spices in this recipe to suit your palate or roast them plain with a little sea salt.

1 (15-ounce) can sodium-free chickpeas, rinsed and dried

2 tablespoons olive oil

1 teaspoon ground cumin

¼ teaspoon smoked paprika

¼ teaspoon sea salt

Pinch cayenne pepper

1. Preheat the oven to 425°F. Line a baking sheet with aluminum foil and set aside.

2. In a large bowl, combine the chickpeas, olive oil, cumin, paprika, sea salt, and cayenne pepper. Toss until the chickpeas are well coated.

3. Spread the chickpeas on the prepared baking sheet. Place in the preheated oven and roast for about 30 minutes, stirring occasionally, or until golden.

4. Cool the chickpeas completely. Refrigerate in a sealed container for up to 1 week.

(Per Serving) Calories: 191; Total Fat: 10g; Saturated Fat: 1g; Carbohydrates: 17g; Fiber: 5g; Protein: 8g

Grilled Carrots with Herbs

SERVES 4 / PREP: 5 MINUTES / COOK: 10 MINUTES

Side dishes do not have to be elaborate to be spectacular. A little oil, a humble root vegetable, and some fresh herbs are all you need to accompany any main course. Carrots get sweeter and their texture has an interesting chewiness at the ends when grilled. If you do not have a grill, broil the carrots in the oven for 10 minutes, turning them several times to get all sides evenly cooked.

1 pound carrots, quartered lengthwise

2 teaspoons olive oil

1 teaspoon chopped fresh dill

1 teaspoon chopped fresh thyme

Sea salt

Freshly ground pepper

1. Preheat the grill (or broiler) to medium.

2. In a large bowl, toss together the carrots, olive oil, dill, and thyme. Season with sea salt and pepper.

3. Grill the carrots for about 10 minutes, turning to cook all sides, until they are crisp-tender and lightly charred. Serve.

PHASE 1: (Per Serving) Calories: 68; Total Fat: 2g; Saturated Fat: 0g; Carbohydrates: 12g; Fiber: 3g; Protein: 1g

PHASE 2: (Per Serving) Calories: 69; Total Fat: 2g; Saturated Fat: 0g; Carbohydrates: 12g; Fiber: 3g; Protein: 1g

PHASE 2 TIP: Add 1 tablespoon of raw apple cider vinegar to the carrots along with the olive oil and herbs.

Succotash

SERVES 4 / PREP: 10 MINUTES / COOK: 20 MINUTES

This is not a traditional succotash with corn, but the tomatoes, spices, herbs, and beans put this dish in a similar category. Chopped zucchini and sweet potato would also be tasty additions. Succotash can be made ahead and popped in the oven to reheat before serving.

1 tablespoon olive oil

1 small sweet onion, chopped

1 teaspoon minced garlic

2 large tomatoes, chopped

1 cup canned navy beans, rinsed

½ teaspoon ground cumin

¼ teaspoon sea salt

Pinch freshly ground black pepper

2 tablespoons julienned fresh basil

1. Place a large saucepan over medium heat and add the olive oil. Add the onion and garlic and sauté for about 4 minutes, or until translucent.

2. Stir in the tomatoes, navy beans, cumin, sea salt, and pepper. Bring to a simmer. Reduce the heat to low and simmer for 15 minutes to combine the flavors.

3. Top with the basil and serve.

(Per Serving) Calories: 128; Total Fat: 4g; Saturated Fat: 1g; Carbohydrates: 19g; Fiber: 5g; Protein: 6g

Sesame Broccoli

SERVES 4 / PREP: 10 MINUTES / COOK: 12 MINUTES

Toasted sesame oil has the most incredible smoky, rich fragrance when heated, which transfers to the broccoli in this recipe. The water added during sautéing steams the broccoli while it cooks in the oil, ensuring a quick preparation time and tender florets. If the florets are smaller than about 2 inches across, decrease the cooking time to 5 to 6 minutes.

1 tablespoon toasted
  sesame oil

1 teaspoon grated
  peeled ginger

½ teaspoon minced garlic

2 broccoli heads, cut into
  small florets

2 tablespoons water

2 tablespoons
  sesame seeds

1. Place a large skillet over medium heat and add the sesame oil. Sauté the ginger and garlic for about 2 minutes, or until fragrant.

2. Add the broccoli florets and water. Sauté for about 10 minutes, or until the broccoli is crisp-tender.

3. Top with sesame seeds and serve.

PHASE 1: (Per Serving) Calories: 104; Total Fat: 6g; Saturated Fat: 1g; Carbohydrates: 10g; Fiber: 4g; Protein: 5g

PHASE 2: (Per Serving) Calories: 105; Total Fat: 6g; Saturated Fat: 1g; Carbohydrates: 10g; Fiber: 4g; Protein: 5g

PHASE 2 TIP: Add 1 tablespoon of raw apple cider vinegar to the broccoli and water.

Coconut Quinoa

SERVES 4 / PREP: 5 MINUTES / COOK: 25 MINUTES

Quinoa is an ancient grain that was cultivated as a staple food thousands of years ago in pre-Columbian civilizations. This seed even had an entire year, 2013, dedicated to it by the Food and Agricultural Organization of the United Nations in tribute to its high nutrition content. Quinoa is packed with antioxidants, phytonutrients, heart-healthy fats, and minerals.

1 tablespoon olive oil

1 small sweet onion, finely chopped

2 teaspoons minced garlic

2 cups unsweetened coconut milk

1 cup quinoa, rinsed

2 teaspoons chopped fresh thyme

Sea salt

¼ cup slivered almonds

¼ cup unsweetened shredded coconut

1. Place a large saucepan over medium heat and add the olive oil. Add the onion and garlic and sauté for about 4 minutes, or until soft.

2. Add the coconut milk and quinoa to the pan. Bring to a boil and reduce the heat to low. Simmer for about 20 minutes, covered, stirring occasionally, until tender.

3. Stir in the thyme and season with sea salt. Top with the almonds and coconut and serve.

PHASE 1: (Per Serving) Calories: 303; Total Fat: 15g; Saturated Fat: 7g; Carbohydrates: 34g; Fiber: 6g; Protein: 8g

PHASE 2: (Per Serving) Calories: 323; Total Fat: 15g; Saturated Fat: 7g; Carbohydrates: 40g; Fiber: 7g; Protein: 8g

PHASE 2 TIP: Add 1 pear, cored and chopped, to the quinoa with the onion.

Roasted Seasonal Veggies

SERVES 4 / PREP: 20 MINUTES / COOK: 45 MINUTES

Use this recipe as a guideline for your own vegetable creations year-round as different vegetables come into season. Try asparagus or green beans in the spring, beets or fennel in the summer, pumpkin or turnips in the fall, and leeks or sweet potatoes in the winter. Most vegetables are delightful when roasted in the oven with a touch of olive oil and a bit of sea salt.

1 eggplant, cut into 1-inch chunks

2 medium zucchini, halved lengthwise and sliced

1 red bell pepper, diced

1 red onion, diced

2 tablespoons olive oil

1 teaspoon chopped fresh thyme

½ teaspoon sea salt

1. Preheat the oven to 350°F. Line a baking sheet with parchment paper and set aside.

2. In a large bowl, toss together the eggplant, zucchini, bell pepper, onion, olive oil, thyme, and sea salt.

3. Transfer the vegetables to the prepared baking sheet and spread them out. Place in the preheated oven and roast for about 45 minutes, or until tender and lightly browned. Serve.

PHASE 1: (Per Serving) Calories: 125; Total Fat: 8g; Saturated Fat: 1g; Carbohydrates: 15g; Fiber: 6g; Protein: 3g

PHASE 2: (Per Serving) Calories: 126; Total Fat: 8g; Saturated Fat: 1g; Carbohydrates: 15g; Fiber: 6g; Protein: 3g

PHASE 2 TIP: Toss 1 tablespoon of raw apple cider vinegar with the other ingredients before roasting.

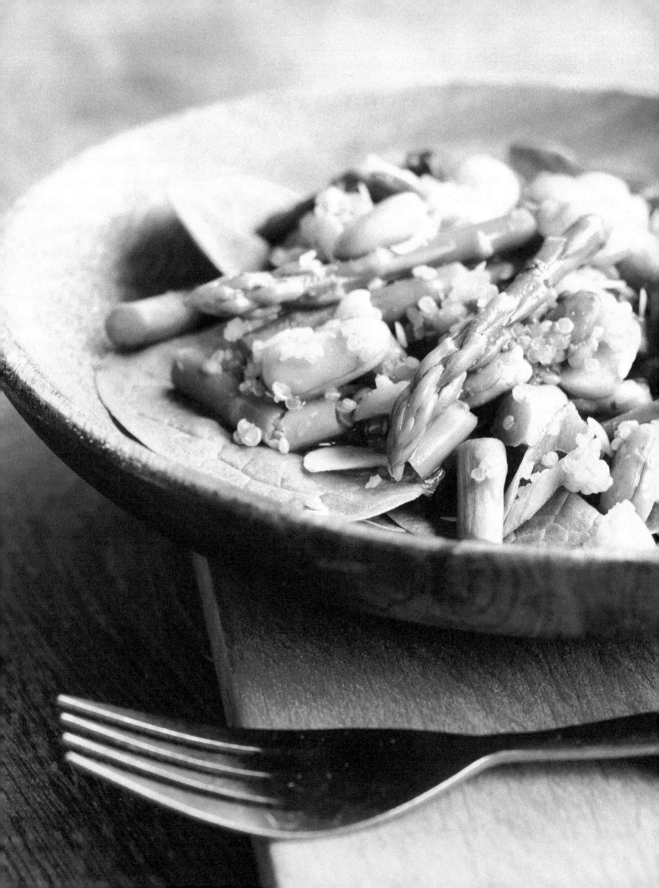

Chapter 4

Soups, Salads, and Sandwiches

Curried Cauliflower Soup

SERVES 4 / PREP: 20 MINUTES / COOK: 35 MINUTES

Puréed cauliflower has a velvety, thick texture, so it makes a marvelous base for luscious creamy soups. Cauliflower is also an excellent source of vitamins C and K, as well as phytonutrients that can help fight cancer and detox the body. Look for a head of creamy white, tightly packed florets surrounded by bright-green, crisp leaves. Avoid vegetables that are look dull or have moldy spots.

1 teaspoon olive oil

1 small sweet onion, chopped

2 teaspoons minced garlic

1 teaspoon grated peeled ginger

1 head cauliflower, cut into small florets

1 sweet potato, peeled and chopped

4 cups chicken broth

1 (14-ounce) can full-fat unsweetened coconut milk

1 tablespoon curry powder

Sea salt

2 tablespoons chopped fresh cilantro

1. Place a large saucepan over medium heat and add the olive oil. Add the onion, garlic, and ginger and sauté for about 4 minutes, or until softened.

2. Stir in the cauliflower, sweet potato, chicken broth, coconut milk, and curry powder, and bring to a boil. Reduce the heat to low and simmer the soup for about 30 minutes, or until the vegetables are tender.

3. Using an immersion blender, a blender, or a food processor, purée the soup until smooth. (If using a blender or food processor, blend the hot soup in small batches.)

4. Season with sea salt. Top with the cilantro and serve.

PHASE 1: (Per Serving) Calories: 317; Total Fat: 26g; Saturated Fat: 21g; Carbohydrates: 21g; Fiber: 6g; Protein: 6g

PHASE 2: (Per Serving) Calories: 353; Total Fat: 28g; Saturated Fat: 23g; Carbohydrates: 24g; Fiber: 6g; Protein: 7g

PHASE 2 TIP: Stir ½ cup of Homemade Coconut Yogurt (page 120) into the soup.

French Onion Soup

SERVES 4 / PREP: 10 MINUTES / COOK: 2 HOURS, 35 MINUTES

The most important ingredient needed to create a robust, intensely flavored onion soup is the patience to caramelize the onions correctly. Let the liquid cook out of the onions, and do not cut the slices too thin or they might burn. Also, do not skip the deglazing step (scraping the flavorful brown bits) or you lose the flavor in the bottom of the pan.

2 tablespoons olive oil

2½ pounds sweet onions, halved and cut into ⅛-inch-thick slices

1 teaspoon minced garlic

6 cups Beef Bone Broth (page 54), divided

1 tablespoon chopped fresh thyme

Sea salt

Freshly ground black pepper

1. Place a large saucepan over low heat and add the olive oil. Add the sliced onions and garlic and stir to combine. Cover the pot and let the juices cook out of the onions for 20 minutes, stirring occasionally.

2. Remove the lid and caramelize the onions, stirring frequently with a wooden spoon and cooking for about 1 hour, 30 minutes, or until they are a deep golden brown.

3. Add 1 cup of the beef broth and scrape up the flavorful browned bits from the bottom of the pan.

4. Stir in the remaining 5 cups of broth and the thyme. Increase the heat to medium to bring the soup to a boil. Reduce the heat to low again and simmer for 45 minutes.

5. Season with sea salt and pepper and serve.

PHASE 1: (Per Serving) Calories: 234; Total Fat: 9g; Saturated Fat: 2g; Carbohydrates: 29g; Fiber: 6g; Protein: 9g

PHASE 2: (Per Serving) Calories: 236; Total Fat: 9g; Saturated Fat: 2g; Carbohydrates: 29g; Fiber: 6g; Protein: 9g

PHASE 2 TIP: Add 2 tablespoons of raw apple cider vinegar to the onions while they are caramelizing.

Rich Tomato Soup

SERVES 4 / PREP: 10 MINUTES / COOK: 35 MINUTES

This is not the canned tomato soup that starred in many childhood lunches. This herb-spiked creation is rich and thick with fresh vegetables. If possible, use organic tomatoes on the vine or those you harvest from your own garden to get the strongest tomato flavor. Hothouse tomatoes are often picked green and ripened on the trucks with ethylene gas, resulting in tomatoes with very little actual taste and only pale coloring.

2 teaspoons olive oil

2 celery stalks, diced

1 sweet onion, chopped

1 tablespoon
    minced garlic

10 large tomatoes,
    chopped

4 cups chicken broth

2 tablespoons chopped
    fresh basil

1 teaspoon chopped
    fresh oregano

Sea salt

Fresh ground
    black pepper

1. Place a large pot over medium heat and add the olive oil. Add the celery, onion, and garlic and sauté for about 5 minutes, or until softened.

2. Stir in the tomatoes and chicken broth. Bring to a boil. Reduce the heat to low and simmer for 30 minutes. Remove from the heat.

3. Using an immersion blender, a blender, or a food processor, purée the soup. (If using a blender or food processor, process the hot soup in small batches.)

4. Stir in the basil and oregano. Season with sea salt and pepper and serve.

PHASE 1: (Per Serving) Calories: 108; Total Fat: 3g; Saturated Fat: 0g; Carbohydrates: 17g; Fiber: 5g; Protein: 5g

PHASE 2: (Per Serving) Calories: 182; Total Fat: 3g; Saturated Fat: 1g; Carbohydrates: 31g; Fiber: 8g; Protein: 10g

PHASE 2 TIP: Add 1 cup of navy beans to the soup before puréeing.

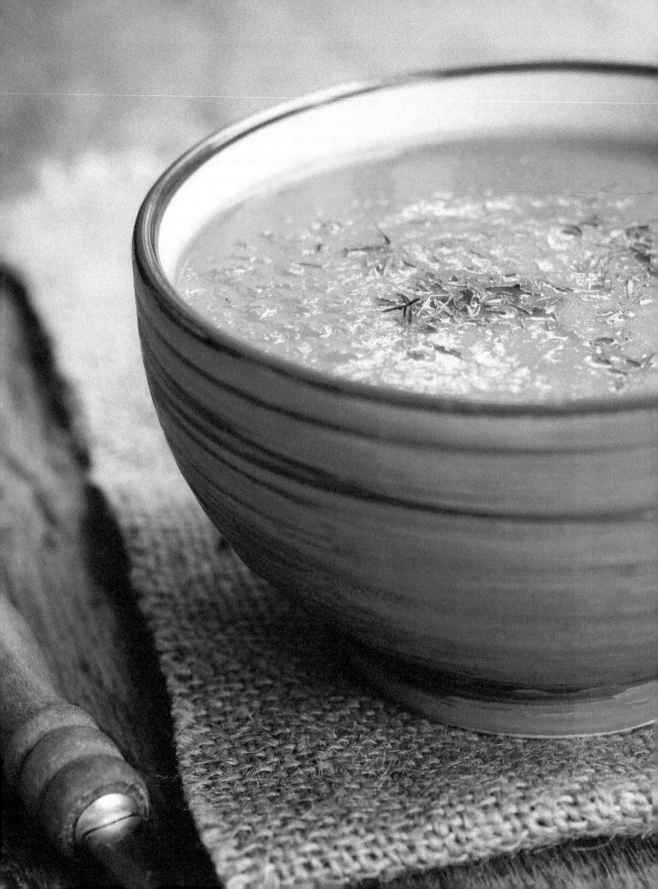

PHASE 1 **PHASE 2**

Creamy Seafood Chowder

SERVES 4 / PREP: 15 MINUTES / COOK: 15 MINUTES

Entire regions stake their tourism reputation on good bowls of fish or clam chowder, so you are in good company when you whip this up at home. Any type of fish, seafood, or shellfish works in chowder, so pick up what's fresh at your local fishmonger or choose a variety that suits your budget. Fish or vegetable broth substitutes well for the chicken broth, if you read the label to be sure there are no additives or gluten in the product.

1 tablespoon olive oil

1 sweet onion, chopped

1 teaspoon minced garlic

1 teaspoon grated
    peeled ginger

4 cups chicken broth

2 celery stalks, chopped

1 carrot, chopped

12 ounces salmon fillets,
    cut into large chunks

15 (16 to 20 count)
    shrimp, peeled,
    deveined,
    and quartered

1 cup canned full-fat
    unsweetened
    coconut milk

1 teaspoon ground cumin

½ teaspoon ground
    turmeric

Pinch red pepper flakes

1 cup shredded kale

Sea salt

Freshly ground
    black pepper

1. Place a large stockpot over medium heat and add the olive oil. Add the onion, garlic, and ginger and sauté for about 4 minutes, or until the vegetables soften.

2. Add the chicken broth, celery, and carrot. Bring to a boil.

3. Stir in the salmon, shrimp, coconut milk, cumin, turmeric, and red pepper flakes. Reduce the heat to low. Simmer the soup for about 5 minutes, or until the fish is cooked through.

4. Stir in the kale. Season with sea salt and pepper and serve immediately.

PHASE 1: (Per Serving) Calories: 419; Total Fat: 26g; Saturated Fat: 15g; Carbohydrates: 12g; Fiber: 3g; Protein: 37g

PHASE 2: (Per Serving) Calories: 473; Total Fat: 29g; Saturated Fat: 17g; Carbohydrates: 16g; Fiber: 3g; Protein: 38g

PHASE 2 TIP: Stir ¾ cup of Homemade Coconut Yogurt (page 120) into the soup along with the kale.

PHASE 1 **PHASE 2**

Chicken-Cabbage Soup

SERVES 4 / PREP: 15 MINUTES / COOK: 45 MINUTES

Chicken soup is regarded as a miracle cure by many people. When you look at the assortment of incredibly nutritious foods in this dish, the idea of food as medicine does not seem far-fetched. Cabbage is a cruciferous vegetable linked to cancer prevention, fennel is packed with immune-boosting phytonutrients, and garlic supports a healthy cardiovascular system. Eat up!

2 tablespoons olive oil

1 sweet onion, chopped

2 teaspoons minced peeled garlic

4 cups shredded green cabbage

2 cups shredded fennel bulb

2 celery stalks, chopped

1 large carrot, chopped

8 cups chicken broth

2 bay leaves

1 cup chopped cooked chicken breast

1 teaspoon chopped fresh thyme

¼ teaspoon sea salt

1. Place a large saucepan over medium heat and add the olive oil. Add the onion and garlic and sauté for about 4 minutes, or until softened.

2. Add the cabbage, fennel, celery, and carrot. Sauté for about 5 minutes, stirring frequently, to soften the cabbage and fennel slightly.

3. Stir in the chicken broth and bay leaves. Bring to a boil. Reduce the heat to low and simmer for about 30 minutes, or until the vegetables are tender.

4. Add the chicken, thyme, and sea salt. Simmer for about 5 minutes more, or until the chicken is heated through.

5. Remove from the heat, discard the bay leaves, and serve.

PHASE 1: (Per Serving) Calories: 186; Total Fat: 9g; Saturated Fat: 2g; Carbohydrates: 14g; Fiber: 4g; Protein: 14g

PHASE 2: (Per Serving) Calories: 250; Total Fat: 10g; Saturated Fat: 2g; Carbohydrates: 26g; Fiber: 9g; Protein: 17g

PHASE 2 TIP: Add 1 cup of cooked navy beans to the soup along with the chicken and thyme.

Beef Bone Broth

MAKES 10 CUPS / PREP: 30 MINUTES / COOK: 25 HOURS + 20 MINUTES COOLING TIME

Bone broth is very nutritious because of the minerals and nutrients that leech from the bones over its long cooking time. Bone broth may seem new, but, in reality, this simple recipe has been around for centuries, especially in Chinese medicine. The addition of raw apple cider vinegar helps draw out the minerals from the bones, so if you are in Phase 2: Rebuild or Phase 3: Revitalize, you will get even more benefit from using this broth in recipes or sipping it as a snack.

3 pounds beef bones

1 sweet onion, peeled and quartered

2 celery stalks, cut into 2-inch pieces

2 carrots, peeled and cut into 1-inch chunks

3 garlic cloves, lightly crushed

2 fresh thyme sprigs

2 bay leaves

1 tablespoon black peppercorns

1 gallon water, plus additional as needed

1. Preheat the oven to 350°F.

2. Place the bones in a baking pan and roast for 30 minutes. Transfer the roasted bones to a large stockpot. Add the onion, celery, carrots, garlic, thyme sprigs, bay leaves, peppercorns, and enough water to cover the bones completely.

3. Put the stockpot over high heat and bring the liquid to a boil. Reduce the heat to low. Cover and simmer for 24 hours. During the first few hours, check the broth every hour and skim off any foam risen to the surface. Remove the pot from the heat and cool for 20 minutes. Remove the bones and discard.

4. Through a fine-mesh sieve, strain the broth and discard the solid bits. Pour the broth into clean jars, put on the lids, and cool completely.

5. Refrigerate the jars for up to 5 days, or freeze for up to 3 months. (If freezing, leave some room for expansion when you pour the broth into the jars.)

PHASE 1: (Per Serving) Calories: 80; Total Fat: 5g; Saturated Fat: 1g; Carbohydrates: 0g; Fiber: 0g; Protein: 4g

PHASE 2: (Per Serving) Calories: 82; Total Fat: 5g; Saturated Fat: 1g; Carbohydrates: 0g; Fiber: 0g; Protein: 4g

PHASE 2 TIP: Add 2 tablespoons of raw apple cider vinegar to the broth.

Crunchy Quinoa-Spinach Salad

SERVES 4 / PREP: 10 MINUTES
COOK: 25 MINUTES + 10 MINUTES COOLING TIME + 2 HOURS CHILLING TIME

Adding turmeric to the cooking liquid with the quinoa creates a glorious sunny hue that complements the other ingredients beautifully. Turmeric is an anti-inflammatory used prominently in Indian and Chinese medicine to treat many ailments. Curcumin is the pigment that gives the spice a bright yellow-orange color and produces an effect in the body similar to fabricated drugs such as ibuprofen and hydrocortisone but without the side effects.

1 teaspoon olive oil

½ small sweet onion, finely diced

1 cup uncooked quinoa, rinsed

2 cups water

1 teaspoon ground turmeric

½ teaspoon ground cumin

1 cup chopped butternut squash

1 cup shredded kale

1 cup halved cherry tomatoes

½ cup roasted shelled unsalted sunflower seeds

1 tablespoon freshly squeezed lemon juice

2 tablespoons chopped fresh parsley

1. Place a medium saucepan over medium heat and add the olive oil. Add the onion and sauté for about 3 minutes, or until soft.

2. Add the quinoa, water, turmeric, cumin, and squash. Bring to a boil. Then, reduce to low heat and cover. Cook the quinoa for 15 minutes. Remove from the heat and let sit for 10 minutes. Fluff the quinoa with a fork and transfer it to a large bowl.

3. Stir in the kale, cherry tomatoes, sunflower seeds, lemon juice, and parsley.

4. Refrigerate the salad for about 2 hours and serve.

PHASE 1: (Per Serving) Calories: 304; Total Fat: 9g; Saturated Fat: 1g; Carbohydrates: 48g; Fiber: 9g; Protein: 11g

PHASE 2: (Per Serving) Calories: 360; Total Fat: 9g; Saturated Fat: 1g; Carbohydrates: 58g; Fiber: 13g; Protein: 16g

PHASE 2 TIP: Add 1 cup of cooked red lentils to the salad.

Shredded Egg–Chard Salad

SERVES 4 / PREP: 15 MINUTES

Consider taking this filling, ingredient-packed salad on your next picnic or to a neighborhood potluck. You probably won't have room for a main course after tucking into the fresh greens, piles of pretty vegetables, salty dill pickle, and protein-packed egg. Make sure the eggs are not freshly laid or you will have difficulty peeling them after they are hardboiled.

FOR THE DRESSING

¼ cup freshly squeezed lemon juice

3 tablespoons olive oil

1 teaspoon raw honey

¼ teaspoon ground mustard

Sea salt

Freshly ground black pepper

FOR THE SALAD

3 cups chopped stemmed Swiss chard

2 cups loosely packed baby spinach

3 large hardboiled eggs, shredded

2 dill pickles, chopped

1 cup green beans, cut into 1-inch pieces

2 radishes, chopped

½ cup walnut halves

TO MAKE THE DRESSING

1. In a small bowl, whisk together the lemon juice, olive oil, honey, and mustard.

2. Season with sea salt and pepper and set aside.

TO MAKE THE SALAD

3. In a large bowl, toss together the Swiss chard, spinach, and the dressing.

4. Divide the greens evenly among 4 plates. Top each salad with a quarter of the eggs, pickles, green beans, radishes, and walnuts. Serve.

(Per Serving) Calories: 265; Total Fat: 23g; Saturated Fat: 3g; Carbohydrates: 8g; Fiber: 3g; Protein: 10g

Lemon-Cucumber Salad

SERVES 2 / PREP: 15 MINUTES

Cucumbers aren't usually considered an exciting salad ingredient because they are used so often in plain iceberg salads in diners and institutional settings. However, cucumbers, which are from the same family as watermelons, are packed with disease-fighting components such as cancer-busting polyphenols. Cucumbers are also very high in phytonutrients and a valuable ingredient for detoxing the body.

FOR THE DRESSING

½ cup raw apple
    cider vinegar

2 tablespoons raw honey

2 tablespoons chopped
    Lacto-Fermented
    Lemons (page 124)

Pinch sea salt

FOR THE SALAD

2 large English
    cucumbers, diced

2 cups blanched
    asparagus spears, cut
    into 1-inch pieces

1 scallion, white and green
    parts, chopped

1 cup cooked quinoa
    (see Tip)

2 tablespoons chopped
    fresh cilantro

2 cups baby spinach

TO MAKE THE DRESSING

1. In a small bowl, whisk together the cider vinegar, honey, and lemon.

2. Season with sea salt and set aside.

TO MAKE THE SALAD

3. In a large bowl, combine the cucumbers, asparagus, scallion, quinoa, and cilantro.

4. Add the dressing and toss to coat.

5. Divide the spinach equally among 4 bowls. Top each serving with a quarter of the cucumber mixture and serve.

(Per Serving) Calories: 157; Total Fat: 2g; Saturated Fat: 0g; Carbohydrates: 32g; Fiber: 4g; Protein: 6g

INGREDIENT TIP: Rinse the quinoa before cooking it to remove the soapy coating called saponins. Saponins can cause digestive upset for some people, so it is best to remove them completely.

Asparagus–Sunflower Seed Salad

SERVES 4 / PREP: 15 MINUTES

Asparagus often appears to be a uniform green color throughout each spear, especially when you blanch it. Peeling thin ribbons of asparagus reveals a subtle shading of color from dark green to a more pastel hue in the center. These multicolored ribbons are stunning tossed with bright-orange carrot in fresh lemon juice.

2 bunches fresh
   asparagus, about
   30 spears

1 carrot

1 tablespoon olive oil

1 scallion, julienned

2 tablespoons freshly
   squeezed lemon juice

1 cup shelled unsalted
   sunflower seeds

2 tablespoons chopped
   fresh thyme

Sea salt

Freshly ground
   black pepper

1. Lay 1 asparagus spear on a cutting board. With a vegetable peeler, shave the spear into long ribbons. Repeat with the remaining spears.

2. Shave the carrot into thin ribbons with the vegetable peeler.

3. In a large bowl, toss the asparagus and carrot ribbons with the olive oil. Add the scallion, lemon juice, sunflower seeds, and thyme. Toss to combine.

4. Season with sea salt and pepper and serve.

PHASE 1: (Per Serving) Calories: 146; Total Fat: 10g; Saturated Fat: 1g; Carbohydrates: 12g; Fiber: 6g; Protein: 7g

PHASE 2: (Per Serving) Calories: 146; Total Fat: 10g; Saturated Fat: 1g; Carbohydrates: 12g; Fiber: 6g; Protein: 7g

PHASE 2 TIP: Substitute raw apple cider vinegar for the lemon juice in this recipe.

Hummus Club Sandwiches

SERVES 4 / PREP: 20 MINUTES

Gluten-free bread suffered from an unfortunate reputation when it first became commercially available because the loaves were heavy and flavorless. With the recognition of widespread celiac issues and the popularity of diets such as Paleo, which shun gluten-containing grains, these breads needed to raise their culinary bar. Gluten-free bread is now quite close to regular bread in appearance and taste, so this sandwich will delight even those who are not on a diet restricting wheat and grain products.

8 gluten-free bread slices, toasted

1 cup homemade hummus (see Tip), divided

4 cooked chicken breast slices, divided

1 cup shredded spinach

1 large tomato, cut into 8 slices

1 large English cucumber, thinly sliced

1. Place 4 slices of the toast on a clean work surface.

2. Spread ¼ cup of the hummus evenly on each piece of bread.

3. Top each with 1 slice of chicken breast, ¼ cup of spinach, 2 tomato slices, and one-quarter of the cucumber slices.

4. Top each with another piece of toast. Cut each sandwich diagonally into 4 pieces and serve.

(Per Serving) Calories: 355; Total Fat: 12g; Saturated Fat: 1g; Carbohydrates: 42g; Fiber: 6g; Protein: 18g

INGREDIENT TIP: Homemade hummus is easy to make. Put 1 (15-ounce) can of water-packed chickpeas (rinsed and drained), 2 tablespoons of tahini (sesame paste), 1 garlic clove, the juice of 1 lemon, 2 tablespoons of olive oil, ½ teaspoon of ground cumin, and a pinch of salt in a blender and process until smooth. You can add a little water if the hummus is too thick for your taste.

Baked Tuna Wraps

SERVES 4 / PREP: 10 MINUTES / COOK: 5 MINUTES

Canned tuna comes in a bewildering range of types including skipjack, albacore, yellow fin, water packed, oil packed, flaked, and solid. You might find yourself standing in the tuna aisle debating for long stretches of time over your choices. The only criterion you need when picking the tuna for this recipe is finding one that is "certified mercury free." Mercury is not recommended on a candida-free diet.

4 gluten-free tortillas

2 cups water-packed tuna, drained

1 scallion, chopped

½ avocado, chopped

¼ cup chopped olives

1 tablespoon freshly squeezed lemon juice

Freshly ground black pepper

1 cup chopped English cucumber

4 ounces alfalfa sprouts

1. Preheat the oven to 350°F.

2. Place the tortillas on a baking sheet.

3. In a medium bowl, stir together the tuna, scallion, avocado, olives, and lemon juice. Season with pepper.

4. Top each tortilla with one-quarter of the tuna mixture.

5. Place the tortillas in the preheated oven and bake for about 5 minutes, or until lightly browned. Remove from the oven.

6. Top each tortilla with ¼ cup of chopped cucumber and 1 ounce of alfalfa sprouts.

7. Wrap the tortillas around the filling and serve.

(Per Serving) Calories: 366; Total Fat: 14g; Saturated Fat: 3g; Carbohydrates: 30g; Fiber: 4g; Protein: 27g

Tabbouleh-Stuffed Pitas

SERVES 2 / PREP: 15 MINUTES

Tabbouleh is a popular Middle Eastern dish that usually features bulgur wheat, but quinoa is a tasty substitution here. This dish is often served wrapped in lettuce leaves as an appetizer, so stuffing it into pitas is not too much of a stretch. If you want a slightly mellower taste, refrigerate the tabbouleh for 1 hour before spooning it into the pitas.

1 cup cooked quinoa

1 cup cooked lentils

2 tablespoons olive oil

Juice of 1 lemon

1 teaspoon minced garlic

2 scallions, finely chopped

1 tomato, diced

½ English cucumber, finely diced

½ cup finely chopped fresh parsley

2 tablespoons chopped fresh mint

4 gluten-free pitas, halved

1 cup Homemade Coconut Yogurt (page 120)

1. In a large bowl, stir together the quinoa, lentils, olive oil, lemon juice, garlic, scallions, tomato, cucumber, parsley, and mint until well mixed.

2. Spoon equal amounts of the quinoa mixture into the 8 pita halves.

3. Top each half with 2 tablespoons of yogurt and serve.

(Per Serving, 2 stuffed pita halves) Calories: 476; Total Fat: 15g; Saturated Fat: 5g; Carbohydrates: 70g; Fiber: 11g; Protein: 17g

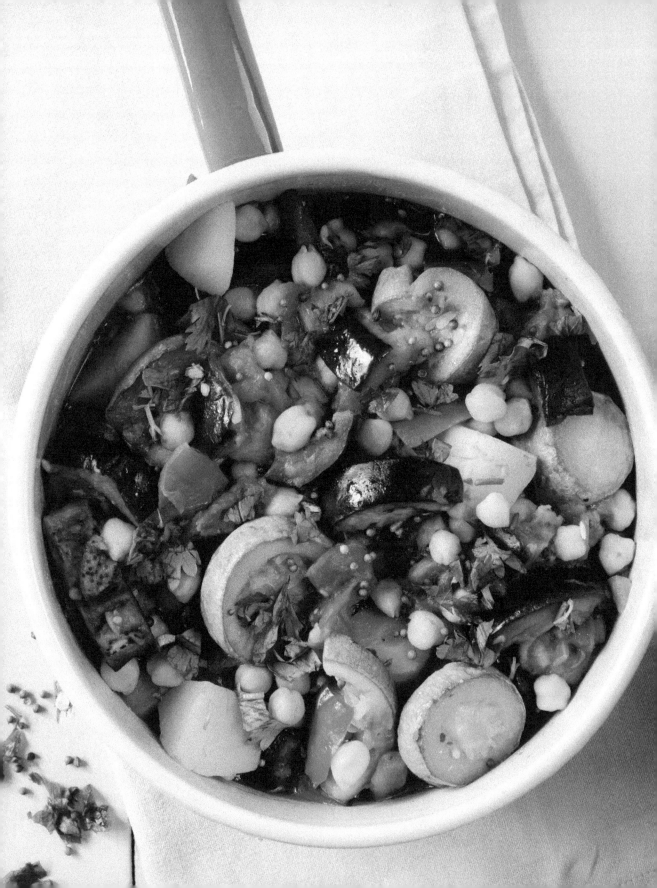

Chapter 5

Meatless Entrées

Artichoke Pesto with Veggie Noodles

SERVES 4 / PREP: 20 MINUTES

Pesto is an all-purpose sauce, condiment, and topper for noodles, fish, or poultry. This versatile concoction can be made from many different ingredients, such as herbs, greens, sun-dried tomatoes, olives, and the artichokes found in this variation. Make a little extra artichoke pesto and keep it in the refrigerator for up to 1 week, for when you need a quick and flavorful addition to your recipes.

2 cups chopped artichoke hearts

½ cup packed fresh basil leaves

½ cup chopped walnuts

2 tablespoons freshly squeezed lemon juice

1 teaspoon minced garlic

Pinch sea salt

Pinch freshly ground black pepper

Pinch red pepper flakes

¼ cup olive oil

2 large zucchini, julienned

2 large carrots, cut with a vegetable peeler into long ribbons

1. In a food processor (or blender), purée the artichoke hearts, basil, walnuts, lemon juice, garlic, sea salt, black pepper, and red pepper flakes.

2. While the processor is running, slowly add the olive oil in a thin stream until the mixture is emulsified.

3. In a large bowl, add the zucchini, carrots, and artichoke pesto and toss to coat. Serve immediately.

PHASE 1: (Per Serving) Calories: 287; Total Fat: 22g; Saturated Fat: 3g; Carbohydrates: 20g; Fiber: 3g; Protein: 9g

PHASE 2: (Per Serving) Calories: 287; Total Fat: 22g; Saturated Fat: 3g; Carbohydrates: 20g; Fiber: 3g; Protein: 9g

PHASE 2 TIP: Substitute raw apple cider vinegar for the lemon juice.

Hummus Burgers

SERVES 4 / PREP: 15 MINUTES + 1 HOUR CHILLING TIME / COOK: 10 MINUTES

Vegetable burgers can also be formed into meatballs rather than patties to create a falafel-like stuffing for pitas. If you make this recipe in burger form, you don't have to stick with traditional burger toppings such as tomato, pickle, and onion. Try sliced avocado, homemade yogurt, pesto, artichokes, and sliced mango to keep things interesting.

1 tablespoon olive oil, divided

1 scallion, finely chopped

¼ cup shredded carrot

½ teaspoon minced garlic

½ teaspoon grated peeled ginger

1 cup cooked chickpeas, rinsed

1 large egg

¼ cup gluten-free bread crumbs plus additional as needed

2 tablespoons chopped fresh parsley

1 teaspoon ground cumin

½ teaspoon ground coriander

Pinch sea salt

1. Place a medium skillet over medium heat and add 1 teaspoon of the olive oil. Sauté the scallion, carrot, garlic, and ginger for about 4 minutes, or until the vegetables soften. Transfer the mixture to a food processor (or blender).

2. Add the chickpeas, egg, bread crumbs, parsley, cumin, coriander, and sea salt. Process until the mixture holds together, adding more bread crumbs if the mixture is too wet. Transfer the mixture to a bowl, cover, and refrigerate for about 1 hour, or until firm.

3. Divide the burger mixture into 4 equal portions. Press them into patties about ½ inch thick.

4. Place a large skillet over medium heat and add the remaining 2 teaspoons of olive oil. Cook the patties for about 3 minutes per side, or until both sides are golden brown. Serve.

(Per Serving) Calories: 168; Total Fat: 8g; Saturated Fat: 2g; Carbohydrates: 18g; Fiber: 4g; Protein: 7g

Quinoa with Heirloom Tomatoes

SERVES 4 / PREP: 15 MINUTES / COOK: 15 MINUTES

This quinoa with heirloom tomatoes is delicious because it is boiled in vegetable broth. If you prefer to use homemade vegetable broth, it's one of the easiest and quickest stocks to make for your recipes. Save the ends of onions, carrots, celery, and scallions along with the peeled skins from root vegetables and place them all in a large pot with fresh herbs, crushed garlic cloves, and black peppercorns. Simmer for 3 to 4 hours and strain. Delicious.

1 teaspoon olive oil

2 teaspoons
minced garlic

2 tablespoons freshly
squeezed lemon juice

2 teaspoons lemon zest

2 cups quinoa, rinsed

4 cups vegetable broth

4 heirloom tomatoes,
each cut into 6 slices

Sea salt

Fresh ground
black pepper

2 tablespoons chopped
fresh cilantro

2 scallions, sliced

1. Place a large saucepan over medium heat and add the olive oil. Add the garlic and sauté for about 1 minute, or until softened.

2. Stir in the lemon juice, lemon zest, quinoa, and vegetable broth. Bring to a boil. Then, reduce the heat to low and simmer for about 15 minutes, or until most of the liquid is absorbed and the quinoa is tender.

3. On each of 4 plates, arrange 6 tomato slices in a circle just inside the rim. Season with sea salt and pepper.

4. Spoon equal amounts of the quinoa over the tomatoes on each plate. Top with cilantro and scallions and serve.

PHASE 1: (Per Serving) Calories: 392; Total Fat: 8g; Saturated Fat: 1g; Carbohydrates: 62g; Fiber: 8g; Protein: 18g

PHASE 2: (Per Serving) Calories: 446; Total Fat: 8g; Saturated Fat: 1g; Carbohydrates: 72g; Fiber: 11g; Protein: 22g

PHASE 2 TIP: Stir 1 cup of cooked red kidney beans into the quinoa.

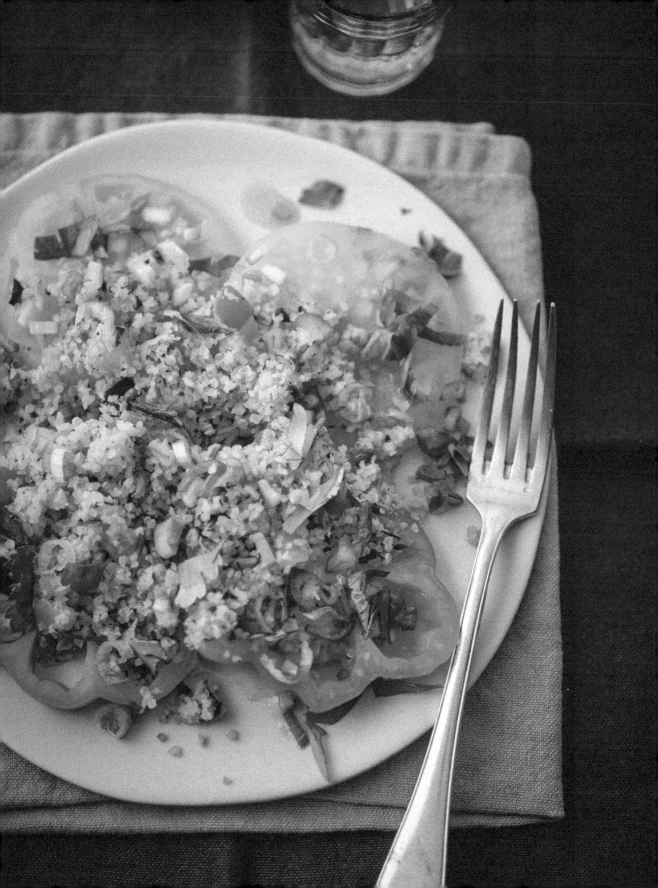

Lentil-Coconut Curry

SERVES 4 / PREP: 15 MINUTES / COOK: 40 MINUTES

Curry is one of the most popular recipes in the world, and there are countless spices, bases, and ingredient combinations for this dish. This curry is not overly hot, although using hot curry powder will certainly turn up the heat. It also has a creamy base rather than a tomato base. The curry powder, squash, red lentils, and carrots create a sunny sauce that makes a dramatic presentation over brown rice or cauliflower rice.

1 tablespoon olive oil

1 small sweet onion, chopped

2 teaspoons minced garlic

2 teaspoons grated peeled ginger

2 cups vegetable broth

1 cup unsweetened coconut milk

2 carrots, diced

½ butternut squash, peeled and diced

1 cup dried red lentils, rinsed and picked over (see Tip)

1 tablespoon curry powder

1 tablespoon raw honey

1 teaspoon chopped fresh thyme

1 cup shredded kale

1. Place a large pot over medium heat and add the olive oil. Add the onion, garlic, and ginger and sauté for about 4 minutes, or until softened.

2. Stir in the vegetable broth, coconut milk, carrots, squash, lentils, curry powder, honey, and thyme. Bring the liquid to a boil. Then, reduce the heat to low and simmer for about 30 minutes, or until the lentils and vegetables are tender and most of the liquid is absorbed.

3. Stir in the kale. Remove the curry from the heat.

4. Serve plain or over brown rice.

(Per Serving) Calories: 445; Total Fat: 19g; Saturated Fat: 14g; Carbohydrates: 58g; Fiber: 21g; Protein: 17g

COOKING TIP: You might be surprised how many tiny stones end up in dried lentils, which is why picking through them is so important. Lentils and other legumes are machine sorted, and since tiny stones have the same general shape as lentils, some make it through.

Ratatouille

SERVES 4 / PREP: 15 MINUTES / COOK: 45 MINUTES

Cuisine that started as peasant food is sometimes the tastiest and most satisfying, because the recipe is meant to use common ingredients and provide sustenance. Ratatouille, a French meal popular in the 1800s, features an abundance of fresh summer vegetables and herbs. Do not overcook this stew because the vegetables should still retain their texture and shape without being mushy.

1 tablespoon olive oil

1 large sweet onion, chopped

2 teaspoons minced garlic

2 medium zucchini, diced

1 small eggplant, diced

1 red bell pepper, sliced thin

½ fennel bulb, cut into 1-inch pieces

2 large tomatoes, chopped

1 cup canned chickpeas, rinsed

½ cup vegetable broth

1 tablespoon freshly squeezed lemon juice

1 tablespoon chopped fresh oregano

1 tablespoon chopped fresh basil

Pinch red pepper flakes

Sea salt

Freshly ground black pepper

1 tablespoon chopped parsley

1. Place a large saucepan over medium-high heat and add the olive oil. Add the onion and garlic and sauté for about 3 minutes, or until softened.

2. Stir in the zucchini, eggplant, bell pepper, and fennel. Sauté for 5 minutes more.

3. Stir in the tomatoes, chickpeas, vegetable broth, and lemon juice. Bring to a boil. Then, reduce the heat to low and simmer for 30 minutes.

4. Stir in the oregano, basil, and red pepper flakes. Simmer for 2 minutes more.

5. Season with sea salt and black pepper. Top with parsley and serve.

PHASE 1: (Per Serving) Calories: 313; Total Fat: 7g; Saturated Fat: 1g; Carbohydrates: 53g; Fiber: 18g; Protein: 14g

PHASE 2: (Per Serving) Calories: 378; Total Fat: 8g; Saturated Fat: 1g; Carbohydrates: 65g; Fiber: 23g; Protein: 18g

PHASE 2 TIP: Stir in 1 cup of cooked navy beans along with the tomatoes.

Summer Vegetable Stew

SERVES 4 / PREP: 10 MINUTES / COOK: 30 MINUTES

Miso is a probiotic food made from fermented soybeans and is often used to balance the microorganisms in the gut. It is packed with antioxidants, protein, and fiber. Certified-organic miso is the best choice if you are concerned about genetically modified (GM) foods; the majority of soybeans produced in the United States are GM products.

1 tablespoon olive oil
1 sweet onion, chopped
2 celery stalks, chopped
1 teaspoon minced garlic
1 sweet potato, diced
2 carrots, diced
2 tomatoes, chopped
1 cup cooked chickpeas
4 cups vegetable broth
1 tablespoon miso
2 cups shredded kale
2 cups cauliflower florets
2 tablespoons chopped
   fresh cilantro
Freshly ground
   black pepper

1. Place a large saucepan over medium heat and add the olive oil. Add the onion, celery, and garlic and sauté for about 5 minutes, or until softened.

2. Stir in the sweet potato, carrots, tomatoes, chickpeas, vegetable broth, and miso. Bring to a boil and cover. Then, reduce the heat to low and simmer for about 15 minutes, or until the vegetables are tender.

3. Stir in the kale and cauliflower and cook for 5 minutes more.

4. Top with the cilantro, season with pepper, and serve.

(Per Serving) Calories: 225; Total Fat: 6g; Saturated Fat: 1g; Carbohydrates: 35g; Fiber: 9g; Protein: 10g

Simple Egg Foo Young

SERVES 2 / PREP: 10 MINUTES / COOK: 15 MINUTES

This delicious omelet is found in several different Chinese cuisines. You can choose to cook individual egg pancakes rather than making a large one and cutting it up. If you make individual pancakes, do 4 in total and stack 2 together on a plate per person.

1 tablespoon toasted sesame oil

1 teaspoon grated peeled ginger

1 teaspoon minced garlic

4 scallions, chopped

2 celery stalks, chopped

1 red bell pepper, chopped

2 cups bean sprouts

6 large eggs, beaten

2 tablespoons chopped fresh cilantro

¼ teaspoon sea salt

1. Place a large skillet over medium heat and add the sesame oil. Add the ginger and garlic and sauté for 1 minute, or until fragrant.

2. Add the scallions, celery, bell pepper, and bean sprouts. Sauté for about 5 minutes, or until the vegetables soften. Spread the vegetables out in an even layer in the skillet.

3. In a small bowl, beat together the eggs, cilantro, and sea salt.

4. Pour the egg mixture over the vegetables in the skillet. Cook for about 5 minutes, or until the eggs are lightly browned, set on the bottom, and look like an omelet. Cut the omelet into quarters and use a spatula to flip the omelet over. Cook for about 3 minutes more, or until the omelet is cooked through.

5. Serve 2 pieces per person.

(Per Serving) Calories: 364; Total Fat: 24g; Saturated Fat: 6g; Carbohydrates: 16g; Fiber: 2g; Protein: 28g

Sun-Dried Tomato Frittata

SERVES 4 / PREP: 15 MINUTES / COOK: 15 MINUTES

Frittatas are like quiche without the crust. The best sun-dried tomatoes you can use are ones you dry yourself in the oven, so you can avoid possible unpleasant additives in store-bought ones. Cut plum tomatoes in half and toss them with olive oil, herbs, sea salt, and pepper. Place them in a single layer on a baking sheet lined with parchment paper and put them into a low-heat oven, about 275°F. Dry the tomatoes slowly for about 12 hours, even overnight, until they are chewy and have an intense tomato flavor. They will stay fresh, refrigerated in a sealed container, for up to 2 weeks.

10 large eggs

½ cup unsweetened almond milk

2 cups shredded spinach

1 tablespoon chopped fresh basil

1 teaspoon chopped fresh oregano

Dash sea salt

Dash freshly ground black pepper

1 teaspoon olive oil

½ sweet onion, chopped

10 oven-dried or sun-dried tomatoes, chopped

1. Preheat the oven to broil.

2. In a large bowl, whisk together the eggs, almond milk, spinach, basil, oregano, sea salt, and pepper until well combined.

3. Place a large ovenproof skillet over medium heat and add the olive oil. Add the onion and sauté for about 3 minutes, or until softened.

4. Add the egg mixture to the skillet. Swirl the skillet, lifting the edges of the cooked egg to allow the uncooked egg to flow underneath. When the frittata is almost set, about 10 minutes, remove it from the heat and sprinkle the top with the tomatoes.

5. Place the frittata in the preheated oven and broil for about 2 minutes, or until the frittata is cooked through and lightly browned on top.

6. Cut into wedges and serve.

PHASE 1: (Per Serving) Calories: 242; Total Fat: 14g; Saturated Fat: 4g; Carbohydrates: 11g; Fiber: 4g; Protein: 19g

PHASE 2: (Per Serving) Calories: 297; Total Fat: 18g; Saturated Fat: 7g; Carbohydrates: 15g; Fiber: 4g; Protein: 20g

PHASE 2 TIP: Whisk ¾ cup of Homemade Coconut Yogurt (page 120) into the egg mixture.

PHASE 1 PHASE 2

Brussels Sprouts–Stuffed Squash

SERVES 2 / PREP: 10 MINUTES / COOK: 55 MINUTES

The pumpkin seeds in this dish add a delightful crunch as well as important nutrients such as zinc, vitamin E, manganese, and phosphorus. For a lovely toasty flavor, roast the shelled seeds in a 300°F oven for 15 minutes, or swirl them in a dry skillet over low heat until they are lightly brown and fragrant. Roasting them any longer can change the fat structure of the seed unfavorably.

1 acorn squash, halved and seeded

1 tablespoon olive oil, divided

2 cups chopped Brussels sprouts

½ cup chopped sweet onion

1 teaspoon minced garlic

1 large tomato, chopped

½ cup shelled pumpkin seeds (pepitas)

1 teaspoon fresh thyme

Sea salt

Freshly ground black pepper

1. Preheat the oven to 400°F. Line a baking sheet with parchment paper.

2. Brush the cut sides of the squash with 1 teaspoon of olive oil. Place the squash, cut-side down, on the baking sheet. Place the baking sheet in the oven and bake for about 30 minutes, or until tender. Remove from the oven and turn the squash over, cut-side up.

3. Place a large skillet over medium heat and add the remaining olive oil. Add the Brussels sprouts, onion, and garlic and sauté for about 6 minutes, or until the vegetables soften. Stir in the tomato, pumpkin seeds, and thyme.

4. From each squash half, scoop out about half of the cooked flesh. Stir the removed flesh into the Brussels sprouts mixture. Season with sea salt and pepper.

5. Spoon the mixture into each squash half and place back in the oven. Bake for 15 minutes and serve.

PHASE 1: (Per Serving) Calories: 201; Total Fat: 12g; Saturated Fat: 2g; Carbohydrates: 22g; Fiber: 5g; Protein: 7g

PHASE 2: (Per Serving) Calories: 289; Total Fat: 12g; Saturated Fat: 2g; Carbohydrates: 36g; Fiber: 12g; Protein: 13g

PHASE 2 TIP: Add 1 cup of cooked red lentils to the Brussels sprouts mixture.

Coconut Pad Thai

SERVES 4 / PREP: 20 MINUTES

Pad Thai usually has a peanut butter–based sauce, and this recipe uses almond butter, which is equally scrumptious. Almond butter can be made at home in a food processor with almonds and a little patience. Purée the almonds for about 20 minutes, until they become a creamy paste rather than just chopped nuts. You can make any kind of nut butter with this technique.

FOR THE SAUCE

¼ cup unsweetened coconut milk

2 tablespoons almond butter

2 tablespoons minced garlic

1 tablespoon chopped fresh cilantro

Dash sea salt

FOR THE VEGETABLES

4 cups shredded napa cabbage

2 large zucchini, cut with a vegetable peeler into long ribbons

2 large carrots, cut with a vegetable peeler into long ribbons

1 red bell pepper, julienned

TO MAKE THE SAUCE

1. In a small bowl, whisk together the coconut milk, almond butter, garlic, cilantro, and sea salt until well combined. Set aside.

TO MAKE THE VEGETABLES

2. In a large bowl, toss together the cabbage, zucchini, carrots, and bell pepper.

3. Add the sauce and toss with tongs to coat. Serve.

PHASE 1: (Per Serving) Calories: 117; Total Fat: 5g; Saturated Fat: 1g; Carbohydrates: 15g; Fiber: 4g; Protein: 7g

PHASE 2: (Per Serving) Calories: 124; Total Fat: 6g; Saturated Fat: 1g; Carbohydrates: 15g; Fiber: 4g; Protein: 7g

PHASE 2 TIP: Whisk 1 teaspoon of miso into the sauce.

Vegetable Nasi Goreng

SERVES 2 / PREP: 10 MINUTES / COOK: 15 MINUTES

Nasi goreng, an Indonesian fried rice, is usually served with a fried egg on top. The golden yolk seeps into the spicy rice, adding richness and a delectable texture. This simple rice creation is often referred to as the national dish of Indonesia because it is served everywhere—from street vendors all the way to fine restaurants.

2 teaspoons toasted sesame oil

2 scallions, chopped

1 teaspoon minced garlic

1 teaspoon grated peeled ginger

1 carrot, chopped

1 red bell pepper, chopped

1 cup chopped cauliflower

2 cups cooked brown rice

2 large eggs, beaten

2 tablespoons chopped fresh cilantro

1. Place a large skillet over medium heat and add the sesame oil. Add the scallions, garlic, and ginger and sauté for about 3 minutes, or until fragrant.

2. Add the carrot, bell pepper, and cauliflower. Sauté for about 6 minutes, or until the vegetables are tender.

3. Stir in the rice and cook for about 4 minutes more, or until heated through.

4. Move the rice mixture to the side of the skillet and add the eggs. Scramble the eggs and then stir them into the rice.

5. Top with the cilantro and serve.

PHASE 1: (Per Serving) Calories: 255; Total Fat: 6g; Saturated Fat: 1g; Carbohydrates: 42g; Fiber: 4g; Protein: 8g

PHASE 2: (Per Serving) Calories: 339; Total Fat: 6g; Saturated Fat: 1g; Carbohydrates: 57g; Fiber: 11g; Protein: 14g

PHASE 2 TIP: Add 1 cup of cooked lentils to the dish with the rice.

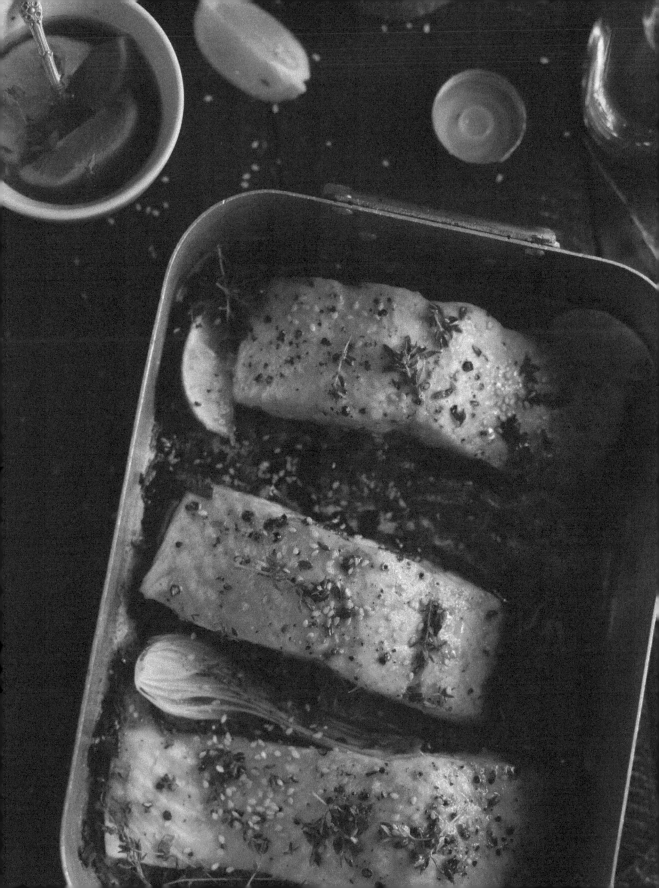

Chapter 6

Fish and Seafood Entrées

Spicy Crab Cakes

SERVES 2 / PREP: 15 MINUTES + 1 HOUR CHILLING TIME / COOK: 10 MINUTES

Good-quality canned and frozen crab is easy to find these days in most grocery stores. Crab is high in nutrients like omega-3 fatty acids, protein, selenium, and chromium, and it's very low in calories. Crab provides many cardiovascular benefits, lowers the risk of some cancers, reduces inflammation, and helps boost the immune system.

1 pound cooked lump crabmeat, drained

¼ cup shredded unsweetened coconut

2 scallions, finely chopped

½ red bell pepper, finely chopped

3 tablespoons coconut flour

1 large egg

1 teaspoon lemon zest

Pinch cayenne pepper

1 tablespoon olive oil

1. In a large bowl, stir together the crabmeat, coconut, scallions, bell pepper, coconut flour, egg, lemon zest, and cayenne pepper until the mixture holds together when pressed.

2. Divide the mixture into 8 portions. Pat them into flat patties about 1 inch thick. Cover and refrigerate for about 1 hour to firm up.

3. Put a large skillet over medium heat and add the olive oil. Add the crab cakes and cook, turning once, for about 4 minutes per side, or until golden. Serve 4 patties per person.

PHASE 1: (Per Serving) Calories: 430; Total Fat: 19g; Saturated Fat: 7g; Carbohydrates: 12g; Fiber: 7g; Protein: 52g

PHASE 2: (Per Serving) Calories: 430; Total Fat: 19g; Saturated Fat: 7g; Carbohydrates: 12g; Fiber: 7g; Protein: 52g

PHASE 2 TIP: Add 1 teaspoon of chopped Lacto-Fermented Lemons (page 124) to the crab mixture.

Baked Coconut Shrimp

SERVES 4 / PREP: 20 MINUTES / COOK: 10 MINUTES

Sweet, plump shrimp coated with toasty golden coconut—what is not to love? Children find this dish charming and fun to eat, especially when you combine it with a tasty dipping sauce. Shrimp is a healthy choice for dinner because it is packed with antioxidants and anti-inflammatories as well as protein, selenium, copper, and vitamin B_{12}. Source your shrimp carefully, looking for wild-caught US shrimp rather than farmed shrimp.

Nonstick cooking spray

½ cup almond flour

1 cup unsweetened shredded coconut

2 large eggs, beaten

1 pound (16 to 20 count) shrimp, deveined and peeled with tails left on

1. Preheat the oven to 450°F. Lightly coat a baking sheet with nonstick cooking spray.

2. In one small shallow bowl, pour in the almond flour; in another small shallow bowl, add the coconut. Put the bowl with the beaten eggs between these 2 bowls.

3. Holding a shrimp by the tail, dredge it in the almond flour. Now dip the shrimp in the egg, shaking off any excess.

4. Finally, dredge the shrimp in the coconut until it is completely coated. Place the coconut-crusted shrimp on the prepared baking sheet. Repeat with the remaining shrimp.

5. Lightly spray the shrimp with cooking spray and place them in the preheated oven. Bake for about 10 minutes, turning once halfway through, until cooked through and the coconut is golden brown. Serve.

(Per Serving) Calories: 441; Total Fat: 28g; Saturated Fat: 15g; Carbohydrates: 10g; Fiber: 6g; Protein: 31g

Seared Scallops with Chickpeas and Greens

SERVES 4 / PREP: 10 MINUTES / COOK: 15 MINUTES

Many home cooks avoid cooking scallops because they assume they are difficult to prepare. Once you become familiar with scallops, issues such as cooking them too long can be avoided easily. The sea scallop is a large scallop—sometimes more than 2 inches in diameter—and the small muscle on the side needs to be removed before cooking. Look for fresh sea scallops that are smooth and uniformly white and avoid those that are frozen because the texture can be unpleasantly mushy.

2 tablespoons olive oil, divided

1½ pounds sea scallops, cleaned and patted dry

Sea salt

Freshly ground black pepper

1 small sweet onion, chopped

½ cup chicken broth

1 cup canned sodium-free chickpeas, rinsed

2 cups kale, shredded

1 tablespoon Kimchi (page 122)

1. Place a large skillet over medium heat and add 1 tablespoon of the olive oil. Lightly season the scallops all over with sea salt and pepper.

2. Add the scallops to the skillet. Sear for about 2 minutes per side, or until opaque and just cooked through. Transfer to a plate and cover loosely with aluminum foil to keep warm.

3. Wipe out the skillet and add the remaining 1 tablespoon of olive oil. Add the onion and sauté for about 3 minutes, or until softened.

4. Add the chicken broth, chickpeas, and kale to the skillet. Cook for about 4 minutes, tossing the greens until they are wilted.

5. Stir in the kimchi and toss to distribute the flavor. Equally divide the mixture among 4 plates, making sure to add all the juices. Top with the scallops and serve.

(Per Serving) Calories: 314; Total Fat: 10g; Saturated Fat: 1g; Carbohydrates: 19g; Fiber: 3g; Protein: 34g

PHASE 1 **PHASE 2**

Mediterranean Fish Stew

SERVES 4 / PREP: 25 MINUTES / COOK: 30 MINUTES

Living on the sparkling waters of the Mediterranean Sea ensures a ready supply of fresh fish and seafood, so seaside countries such as Greece and Italy incorporate these ingredients into many traditional recipes. You can create your own variation with whatever fish is freshest in your area, or maybe you can even catch it yourself.

2 tablespoons olive oil

2 celery stalks, chopped

1 sweet onion, chopped

1 teaspoon minced garlic

2 cups fish broth

3 tomatoes, chopped

2 bay leaves

2 teaspoons chopped
    fresh thyme

2 sweet potatoes, peeled
    and diced

2 parsnips, peeled
    and diced

2 tablespoons chopped
    fresh parsley

½ pound halibut fillet, cut
    into 1-inch pieces

½ pound salmon fillet, cut
    into 1-inch pieces

3 cups shredded
    baby spinach

Sea salt

Freshly ground
    black pepper

1. Place a large stockpot over medium heat and add the olive oil. Add the celery, onion, and garlic and sauté for about 3 minutes, or until softened.

2. Stir in the fish broth, tomatoes, bay leaves, and thyme. Bring to a boil. Reduce the heat to low so the stew simmers.

3. Stir in the sweet potatoes and parsnips. Continue to simmer for about 20 minutes, or until the vegetables are tender.

4. Remove and discard the bay leaves. Stir in the parsley, halibut, and salmon. Simmer for about 5 minutes, or until the fish is cooked through.

5. Stir in the spinach. Season with sea salt and pepper and serve.

PHASE 1: (Per Serving) Calories: 362; Total Fat: 13g; Saturated Fat: 2g; Carbohydrates: 37g; Fiber: 8g; Protein: 29g

PHASE 2: (Per Serving) Calories: 416; Total Fat: 13g; Saturated Fat: 2g; Carbohydrates: 47g; Fiber: 12g; Protein: 33g

PHASE 2 TIP: Add 1 cup of cooked cannellini beans to the stew along with the fish.

Shrimp Skillet with Brown Rice

SERVES 4 / PREP: 20 MINUTES / COOK: 15 MINUTES

If your typical weekday evenings include running out the door again for a child's music lesson or sports game or an evening meeting for work, this recipe might become your go-to choice for a quick, filling meal. Cooked brown rice will stay fresh in the refrigerator for about 5 days and in the freezer for up to 3 months. So, whipping up a big pot of rice at the beginning of the week can save lots of time. Seal the extra rice in plastic freezer bags in the correct amounts for meals later in the week.

1 tablespoon olive oil

½ eggplant, halved lengthwise and cut into ½-inch wedges

½ sweet onion, chopped

1 teaspoon minced garlic

1 pound (16 to 20 count) shrimp, peeled and deveined

2 cups cooked brown rice

1 scallion, cut into thin slices

½ teaspoon ground cumin

½ teaspoon ground coriander

Sea salt

Freshly ground black pepper

2 tablespoons chopped basil

1. Place a large skillet over medium heat and add the olive oil. Add the eggplant, onion, and garlic and sauté for about 6 minutes, or until the vegetables soften. Move the vegetables to the side of the skillet.

2. Add the shrimp and sauté for about 5 minutes, or until opaque. Move the shrimp over with the vegetables.

3. Add the rice, scallion, cumin, and coriander. Cook, stirring, for about 4 minutes, or until the rice is heated through.

4. Season with sea salt and pepper.

5. Scoop the rice onto 4 plates and top each with one-quarter of the vegetables and shrimp. Garnish with the chopped basil and serve.

PHASE 1: (Per Serving) Calories: 360; Total Fat: 7g; Saturated Fat: 1g; Carbohydrates: 43g; Fiber: 4g; Protein: 30g

PHASE 2: (Per Serving) Calories: 424; Total Fat: 7g; Saturated Fat: 1g; Carbohydrates: 55g; Fiber: 9g; Protein: 34g

PHASE 2 TIP: Add 1 cup of navy beans to the dish along with the brown rice.

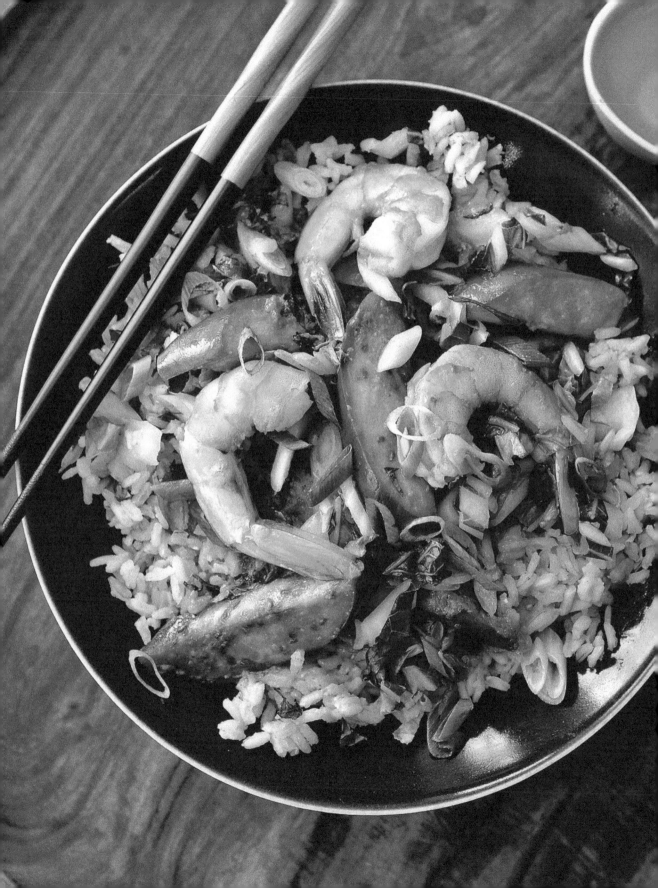

Lemon-Poached Salmon

SERVES 4 / PREP: 10 MINUTES / COOK: 1 HOUR

In this dish, the salmon comes out of its poaching liquid with a delicate, herbal flavor and a hint of citrus. Salmon is an excellent source of omega-3 fatty acid, which supports cardiovascular, nerve, and brain health. Whenever possible, purchase wild-caught salmon because farmed salmon can have contamination issues.

8 cups water

½ cup freshly squeezed lemon juice

1 sweet onion, sliced

1 cup chopped celery greens

1 small carrot, sliced

2 teaspoons chopped fresh dill

2 teaspoons chopped fresh thyme

1 bay leaf

¼ teaspoon sea salt

1 teaspoon black peppercorns

4 (6-ounce) salmon fillets

1. In a large pot set over high heat, combine the water, lemon juice, onion, celery greens, carrot, dill, thyme, bay leaf, sea salt, and peppercorns. Bring to a full boil. Reduce the heat to low and simmer the liquid for 45 minutes.

2. Strain the stock through a sieve into a large skillet set over low heat. Bring to a simmer.

3. Add the salmon and cover the skillet. Simmer for 10 minutes, or until the fish is opaque and just cooked through.

4. Remove the poached salmon carefully and serve.

(Per Serving) Calories: 252; Total Fat: 11g; Saturated Fat: 2g; Carbohydrates: 5g; Fiber: 1g; Protein: 34g

Jerk-Rubbed Halibut

SERVES 4 / PREP: 10 MINUTES / COOK: 10 MINUTES

Jerk seasoning is usually associated with meats or poultry, but it can be just as tasty sprinkled on fish. This Jamaican spice mix can have many different ingredients, although most versions include allspice, also known as pimento berries. The word *jerk* is thought to have derived from the practice of poking holes in the meat or poultry to get the spices to penetrate better.

½ teaspoon garlic powder

¼ teaspoon cayenne pepper

¼ teaspoon onion powder

¼ teaspoon paprika

⅛ teaspoon ground allspice

⅛ teaspoon red pepper flakes

⅛ teaspoon ground cinnamon

4 (6-ounce) halibut fillets

1 tablespoon olive oil

1. In a small bowl, stir together the garlic powder, cayenne pepper, onion powder, paprika, allspice, red pepper flakes, and cinnamon.

2. Sprinkle the fish fillets evenly on both sides with the jerk seasoning.

3. Place a large skillet over medium heat and add the olive oil. Panfry the fish for about 4 minutes per side, or until it is cooked through and browned. Serve.

PHASE 1: (Per Serving) Calories: 172; Total Fat: 5g; Saturated Fat: 1g; Carbohydrates: 1g; Fiber: 0g; Protein: 32g

PHASE 2: (Per Serving) Calories: 263; Total Fat: 11g; Saturated Fat: 6g; Carbohydrates: 7g; Fiber: 0g; Protein: 34g

PHASE 2 TIP: Serve the fish with an herb yogurt sauce made by blending 1 cup of Homemade Coconut Yogurt (page 120) with 1 teaspoon of freshly squeezed lemon juice, 1 teaspoon of chopped cilantro, and 1 teaspoon of chopped basil.

Sesame-Crusted Salmon

SERVES 4 / PREP: 15 MINUTES / COOK: 18 MINUTES

Sesame seeds are one of the oldest items used as a condiment and medicinal aid. They are exceptionally high in calcium, copper, and manganese, which is why they can positively affect rheumatoid arthritis and support healthy respiratory and cardiovascular systems. There is no real difference between the black and white sesame seeds; the black ones still have their hulls. Just use whatever type you have in the pantry.

4 (6-ounce) salmon fillets

¼ teaspoon sea salt

2 tablespoons white sesame seeds

2 tablespoons black sesame seeds

1 tablespoon chopped fresh thyme

1 tablespoon olive oil

¼ cup vegetable stock

1. Preheat the oven to 400°F.

2. Pat the salmon fillets dry with paper towels and season with sea salt. Place the salmon in a baking dish and sprinkle the sesame seeds and thyme over the fillets evenly.

3. Drizzle the salmon with olive oil and pour the vegetable stock into the baking dish.

4. Bake the salmon until just cooked through and the sesame seeds are golden and crispy, 15 to 18 minutes. Serve.

(Per Serving) Calories: 300; Total Fat: 18g; Saturated Fat: 3g; Carbohydrates: 2g; Fiber: 1g; Protein: 34g

Haddock with Cucumber-Mint Salsa

SERVES 4 / PREP: 15 MINUTES / COOK: 10 MINUTES

The various shades of green in this salsa are not hidden by the creamy yogurt, and you might be reminded of tzatziki when you first taste it. The cool flavor of the chopped mint comes from the menthol in the herb. Menthol is a common treatment for digestive issues, colds, flu, and nausea. Mint can also boost immunity and cleanse the blood.

FOR THE SALSA

¼ cup Homemade Coconut Yogurt (page 120)

½ cup grated English cucumber, liquid squeezed out

1 kiwi, peeled and chopped

2 tablespoons chopped fresh mint

1 teaspoon raw honey

FOR THE HADDOCK

2 teaspoons olive oil

4 (5-ounce) haddock fillets, patted dry

Sea salt

Fresh ground black pepper

TO MAKE THE SALSA

1. In a small bowl, stir together the yogurt, cucumber, kiwi, mint, and honey until well mixed. Set aside.

TO MAKE THE HADDOCK

2. Place a large skillet over medium heat and add the olive oil.

3. Season the haddock lightly with sea salt and pepper.

4. Panfry the haddock for about 5 minutes per side, turning once, or until just cooked through.

5. Top with the cucumber-mint salsa and serve.

(Per Serving) Calories: 235; Total Fat: 6g; Saturated Fat: 2g; Carbohydrates: 8g; Fiber: 1g; Protein: 36g

COOKING TIP: Mint is often sold in large bunches so you might have some left over. Chop the entire bunch and scatter the pieces on a parchment-lined baking sheet. Place the sheet in the freezer and, when the mint is frozen, transfer it to a resealable plastic bag. If you press out all the air, the mint can be used straight from the freezer for up to 3 months.

Coconut-Crusted Sea Bass

SERVES 4 / PREP: 10 MINUTES / COOK: 15 MINUTES

Sea bass is a generic term for several types of fish, some of which, like Chilean sea bass, are not bass at all. When choosing the fish for this meal, stay away from Chilean sea bass because it is high in mercury.

4 (5-ounce) boneless white or striped sea bass fillets, patted dry

Sea salt

Freshly ground black pepper

1 cup shredded unsweetened coconut

1 tablespoon olive oil

Lime wedges, for garnish

1. Preheat the oven to 400°F. Line a baking sheet with parchment paper and set aside.

2. Lightly season the sea bass with sea salt and pepper.

3. Place the coconut on a plate. Press both sides of the fish fillets into the coconut to coat, and place the fish on the prepared baking sheet. Repeat with the remaining fillets.

4. Drizzle the coconut-crusted fish with the olive oil.

5. Place the fish in the preheated oven and bake for about 15 minutes, or until the coconut is golden and the fish flakes easily when lightly pressed with a fork. Serve with the lime wedges.

(Per Serving) Calories: 178; Total Fat: 9g; Saturated Fat: 6g; Carbohydrates: 3g; Fiber: 2g; Protein: 18g

Ginger-Salmon Burgers

SERVES 4 / PREP: 10 MINUTES + 1 HOUR CHILLING TIME / COOK: 10 MINUTES

Friday night dinners in the 1970s often featured soggy, tasteless fish burgers drenched in ketchup to make them palatable. If you stay away from fish burgers because of bad impressions, these moist, flavorful patties will be a wonderful surprise. The fresh chopped salmon is the ingredient that makes the difference and elevates these burgers to a fine-dining level.

1 (1-pound) salmon
   fillet, chopped

1 scallion, chopped

1 tablespoon chopped
   fresh cilantro

1 tablespoon coconut
   flour, plus more
   as needed

1 teaspoon grated
   peeled ginger

¼ teaspoon sea salt

1 tablespoon olive oil

1. In a large bowl, mix together the salmon, scallion, cilantro, coconut flour, ginger, and sea salt until the mixture is well combined and holds together when pressed. Add more coconut flour if the mixture is too wet.

2. Form the salmon mixture into 4 patties, each about ½ inch thick. Place them on a plate, cover, and refrigerate for 1 hour to firm up.

3. Place a large skillet over medium heat and add the olive oil. Panfry the patties for about 10 minutes, turning once halfway through, until golden and lightly crispy but still slightly pink in the center. Serve.

PHASE 1: (Per Serving) Calories: 192; Total Fat: 11g; Saturated Fat: 2g; Carbohydrates: 2g; Fiber: 1g; Protein: 23g

PHASE 2: (Per Serving) Calories: 192; Total Fat: 11g; Saturated Fat: 2g; Carbohydrates: 2g; Fiber: 1g; Protein: 23g

PHASE 2 TIP: Add 1 teaspoon of chopped Lacto-Fermented Lemons (page 124) to the salmon mixture.

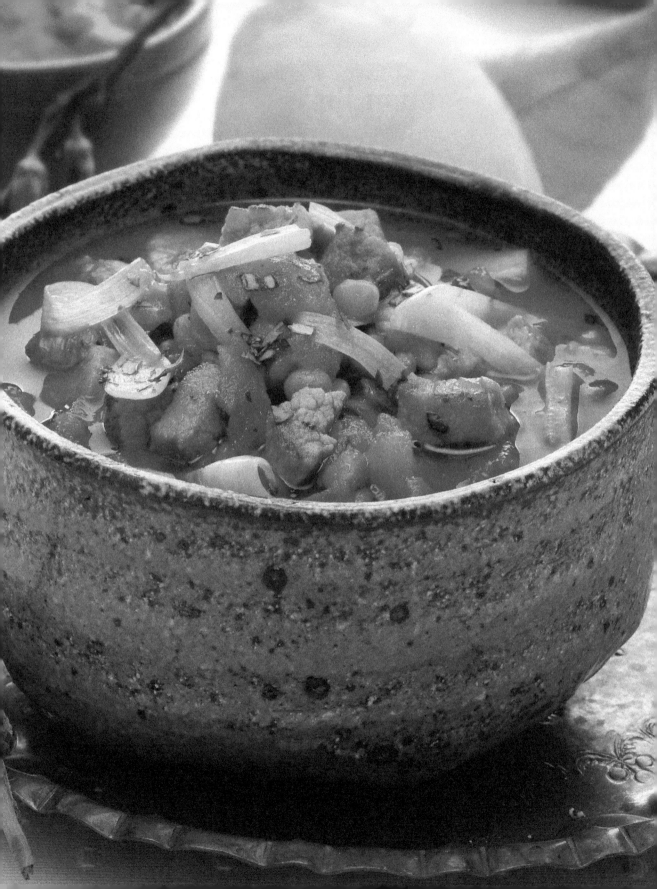

Chapter 7

Meat and Poultry Entrées

Golden Chicken Fingers

SERVES 4 / PREP: 20 MINUTES / COOK: 15 MINUTES

If you have kids in your home, chicken fingers are probably on the menu as many times as they can convince you to make or purchase them. There is something fun and festive about these golden juicy chicken strips, especially if served with a dipping sauce. Try puréed roasted red pepper, or mango with a hint of spice, or a sugar-free tomato sauce for a change.

¼ cup fine almond flour

¼ cup unsweetened coconut milk

1 large egg

1 cup almond meal

2 (8-ounce) boneless skinless chicken breasts, cut lengthwise into 6 strips, patted dry

Olive oil cooking spray

1. Preheat the oven to 400°F. Line a baking sheet with parchment paper and set aside.

2. Place the almond flour in a small shallow bowl and set aside. In another small, shallow bowl, whisk together the coconut milk and egg, and set aside. Put the almond meal into a third small, shallow bowl.

3. Dredge 1 chicken strip in the almond flour, dip it into the coconut milk mixture, and finally, dredge it in the almond meal until completely coated. Place on the prepared baking sheet. Repeat this process with the remaining chicken strips.

4. Lightly spray the coated chicken with cooking spray. Place in the preheated oven and bake, turning once halfway through, for about 15 minutes, or until golden and serve.

PHASE 1: (Per Serving) Calories: 489; Total Fat: 28g; Saturated Fat: 6g; Carbohydrates: 14g; Fiber: 3g; Protein: 35g

PHASE 2: (Per Serving) Calories: 507; Total Fat: 29g; Saturated Fat: 7g; Carbohydrates: 15g; Fiber: 3g; Protein: 35g

PHASE 2 TIP: Replace the egg in the breading process with 2 tablespoons of Homemade Coconut Yogurt (page 120).

Chicken Cacciatore

SERVES 6 / PREP: 30 MINUTES / COOK: 35 MINUTES

Chicken cacciatore is often made with chicken thighs instead of breasts because the dark meat tastes richer with all the vegetables and herbs. However, this version contains less fat. Whenever possible, use the center portion of the celery bunch and include the greens for added flavor. Celery is an excellent source of vitamin C, calcium, magnesium, and potassium. It can help fight cancer, lower blood pressure, and boost the immune system.

2 tablespoons olive oil

4 (6-ounce) boneless skinless chicken breasts, cut into 1½-inch chunks

1 sweet onion, chopped

2 teaspoons minced garlic

3 celery stalks, chopped

1 red bell pepper, chopped

6 large tomatoes, chopped

2 cups cooked cannellini beans, rinsed

6 pickled artichoke hearts, quartered

5 sun-dried tomatoes, coarsely chopped

½ cup chicken broth

¼ cup chopped fresh basil

2 tablespoons chopped fresh oregano

Pinch red pepper flakes

Sea salt

Freshly ground black pepper

Brown rice or gluten-free pasta, for serving

1. In large saucepan set over medium heat, heat the olive oil. Add the chicken and sauté for about 7 minutes, or until lightly browned and almost cooked through. With a slotted spoon, transfer the chicken to a plate and set aside.

2. Add the onion and garlic to the pan. Sauté for about 4 minutes, or until the onion is translucent.

3. Stir in the celery and bell pepper. Sauté for 2 minutes.

4. Pour the chicken back in the pan and add the tomatoes, cannellini beans, artichoke hearts, sun-dried tomatoes, chicken broth, basil, oregano, and red pepper flakes. Bring the mixture to a boil. Then, reduce the heat to low and simmer for about 20 minutes, or until the chicken is cooked through and the flavors blend.

5. Season with sea salt and black pepper. Serve over brown rice or gluten-free pasta.

(Per Serving) Calories: 473; Total Fat: 14g; Saturated Fat: 3g; Carbohydrates: 44g; Fiber: 19g; Protein: 46g

Roasted Chicken with Herbs

SERVES 6 / PREP: 15 MINUTES
COOK TIME: 1 HOUR, 30 MINUTES + 15 MINUTES RESTING TIME

Roasted chicken makes a spectacular presentation and is one of the simplest meals to create with very little preparation time. You can pop the chicken into the oven in a roasting pan and, in just over an hour, have an elegant meal with an accompanying side dish on the table. When selecting chicken, get one labeled "roaster" because this means it is less than 8 months old and still tender.

1 (4-pound) whole roasting chicken

1 teaspoon sea salt, divided

4 shallots, peeled and lightly crushed

4 fresh thyme sprigs

2 fresh rosemary sprigs

1 tablespoon olive oil

½ teaspoon freshly ground black pepper

1. Preheat the oven to 350°F.

2. Wash the chicken with cold water, inside and out, and pat it completely dry with paper towels.

3. Place the chicken in a baking dish, and lightly salt the cavity with ½ teaspoon of salt. Place the shallots, thyme, and rosemary in the cavity. Brush the chicken skin all over with the olive oil, and season the skin with the remaining salt and the pepper.

4. Roast the chicken until it is golden brown and cooked through (internal temperature of 185°F), about 1 hour and 30 minutes.

5. Remove the chicken from the oven, and let it sit for 15 minutes before removing the shallots, thyme, and rosemary from the cavity.

6. Carve the chicken, and serve.

PHASE 1: (Per Serving) Calories: 174; Total Fat: 6g; Saturated Fat: 1g; Carbohydrates: 3g; Fiber: 0g; Protein: 25g

PHASE 2: (Per Serving) Calories: 176; Total Fat: 6g; Saturated Fat: 1g; Carbohydrates: 3g; Fiber: 0g; Protein: 25g

PHASE 2 TIP: Add 2 tablespoons of raw apple cider vinegar to the pan along with the juices from the chicken.

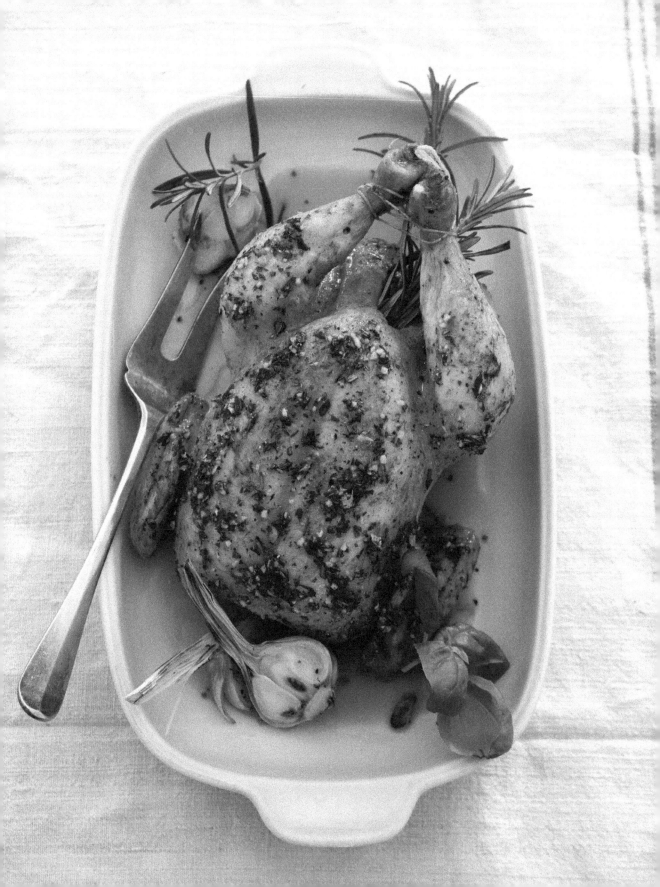

Coconut-Butter Chicken

SERVES 4 / PREP: 15 MINUTES / COOK: 25 MINUTES

Butter chicken is one of the better-known Indian dishes in the world and is a delicious staple on many Indian restaurant menus. This version comes from northern India and features a spiced tomato sauce spiked with creamy yogurt. Even without butter, it still tastes very similar to the traditional recipe.

1 tablespoon olive oil

3 (6-ounce) boneless skinless chicken breasts, cut into 1-inch chunks

1 scallion, chopped

1 tablespoon minced garlic

1 tablespoon grated peeled ginger

1 tablespoon freshly squeezed lemon juice

1 teaspoon garam masala

1 teaspoon ground cumin

½ teaspoon fenugreek

Pinch red pepper flakes

1 tomato, chopped

1 cup unsweetened coconut milk

1 cup Homemade Coconut Yogurt (page 120)

Sea salt

Freshly ground black pepper

2 tablespoons chopped fresh cilantro

Brown rice, for serving

1. Place a large saucepan over medium heat and add the olive oil. Add the chicken and sauté for about 5 minutes, or until almost cooked through. With a slotted spoon, transfer the chicken to a plate and set aside.

2. Add the scallion, garlic, and ginger to the saucepan. Sauté for 3 minutes.

3. Stir in the lemon juice, garam masala, cumin, fenugreek, and red pepper flakes. Sauté for about 1 minute, or until fragrant.

4. Stir in the tomato and simmer for 1 minute more.

5. Add the coconut milk and yogurt. Bring the sauce to a boil. Reduce the heat to low and simmer for 7 minutes.

6. Add the chicken back to the sauce with any drippings on the plate. Continue to simmer for 5 minutes more.

7. Season with sea salt and black pepper. Top with the cilantro and serve over brown rice.

(Per Serving) Calories: 390; Total Fat: 28g; Saturated Fat: 9g; Carbohydrates: 10g; Fiber: 1g; Protein: 40g

INGREDIENT TIP: The taste of fenugreek can be compared to toasted or burnt celery. Do not omit this spice, because it is what gives butter chicken its distinctive flavor.

Turkey with Lentils, Cranberries, and Mint

SERVES 4 / PREP: 15 MINUTES / COOK: 10 MINUTES

Turkey is sometimes overlooked, except when you need a gigantic bird to stuff and serve on a holiday. Cuts of turkey such as breasts, legs, and thighs can be found in most grocery store cold cases so you don't have to wait for Thanksgiving to enjoy this nutritious food. Turkey is a good source of protein, potassium, zinc, and iron, and two-thirds of its fat content is unsaturated.

FOR THE SAUCE

2 tablespoons freshly squeezed lime juice

1 tablespoon olive oil

½ teaspoon ground cinnamon

¼ teaspoon ground coriander

¼ teaspoon ground cumin

Pinch freshly ground black pepper

FOR THE LENTILS

1 teaspoon olive oil

1 scallion, white and green parts, chopped

3 cups cooked lentils, rinsed and drained

1 cup peas

1 cup chopped cooked turkey breast

1 carrot, shredded

1 cup shredded kale

½ cup dried cranberries

½ cup shelled unsalted sunflower seeds

1 tablespoon chopped fresh mint

TO MAKE THE SAUCE

1. In a small bowl, stir together the lime juice, olive oil, cinnamon, coriander, cumin, and pepper. Set aside.

TO MAKE THE LENTILS

2. Place a large saucepan over medium heat and add the olive oil. Add the scallion and sauté for about 2 minutes, or until tender.

3. Add the lentils, peas, turkey, carrot, and kale. Sauté for about 6 minutes, or until heated through. Remove from the heat.

4. Stir in the sauce, cranberries, sunflower seeds, and mint. Serve.

(Per Serving) Calories: 455; Total Fat: 10g; Saturated Fat: 1g; Carbohydrates: 59g; Fiber: 26g; Protein: 34g

Turkey Meatloaf

SERVES 4 / PREP: 10 MINUTES / COOK: 55 MINUTES + 10 MINUTES RESTING TIME

Meatloaf can include a plethora of difficult-to-find ingredients or be as simple as seasoning, meat, bread crumbs, and an egg. This recipe is obviously the simple kind, but it is certainly not lacking in flavor. You might want to whip up two of these savory meatloaves so you have extra for lunch the next day.

1 teaspoon olive oil

½ small sweet onion, finely chopped

1 teaspoon minced garlic

½ teaspoon grated peeled ginger

1 pound lean ground turkey

1 large egg

1 carrot, grated

½ cup almond meal

Pinch sea salt

Pinch freshly ground black pepper

1. Preheat the oven to 350°F.

2. Place a small skillet over medium heat and add the olive oil. Sauté the onion, garlic, and ginger for about 3 minutes, or until tender. Transfer the vegetables to a large bowl.

3. Add the turkey, egg, carrot, almond meal, sea salt, and pepper. With clean hands, mix the ingredients well. Pack the mixture into an 8-by-4-inch loaf pan, leaving some room around the sides. Place the pan in the preheated oven and bake for about 50 minutes, or until cooked through and golden on top. Remove from the oven and let the meatloaf rest for 10 minutes.

4. Drain off any visible grease and serve.

PHASE 1: (Per Serving) Calories: 289; Total Fat: 14g; Saturated Fat: 4g; Carbohydrates: 15g; Fiber: 2g; Protein: 26g

PHASE 2: (Per Serving) Calories: 325; Total Fat: 15g; Saturated Fat: 5g; Carbohydrates: 19g; Fiber: 3g; Protein: 28g

PHASE 2 TIP: Add ½ cup of puréed sodium-free chickpeas to the meatloaf mixture instead of the egg.

North African Lamb Stew

SERVES 4 / PREP: 20 MINUTES / COOK: 2 HOURS, 30 MINUTES

Lamb is can be found year-round, although spring lamb is still considered by many chefs to be the best. If your budget permits, and you have access to a wide assortment of ingredients, look for 100 percent grass-fed organic lamb. This designation ensures that the lamb was most likely humanely raised and is free of antibiotics.

2 tablespoons olive oil

1½ pounds lamb shoulder, trimmed of visible fat, and cut into 1-inch chunks

1 sweet onion, chopped

2 teaspoons minced garlic

1 teaspoon grated peeled ginger

1 teaspoon ground cinnamon

½ teaspoon ground turmeric

¼ teaspoon ground cloves

2 cups Beef Bone Broth (page 54), or purchased beef broth

2 tomatoes, chopped

2 celery stalks, diced

2 cups chopped butternut squash

2 cups cauliflower florets

2 tablespoons chopped fresh parsley

1. Preheat the oven to 300°F.

2. Place a large ovenproof skillet over medium heat and add the olive oil. Add the lamb and sauté for about 4 minutes.

3. Stir in the onion, garlic, ginger, cinnamon, turmeric, and cloves. Sauté for 5 minutes more.

4. Add the beef broth, tomatoes, celery, and squash. Bring to a boil. Then, cover the skillet and place it in the preheated oven. Braise the stew for about 2 hours, stirring occasionally, until the lamb is very tender.

5. Remove the stew from the oven and stir in the cauliflower. Return the stew to the oven for about 10 minutes, or until the cauliflower is tender.

6. Sprinkle with the parsley and serve.

PHASE 1: (Per Serving) Calories: 446; Total Fat: 20g; Saturated Fat: 6g; Carbohydrates: 16g; Fiber: 3g; Protein: 51g

PHASE 2: (Per Serving) Calories: 482; Total Fat: 22g; Saturated Fat: 7g; Carbohydrates: 18g; Fiber: 4g; Protein: 51g

PHASE 2 TIP: Stir in ½ cup of Homemade Coconut Yogurt (page 120) when the stew is ready to serve.

Grilled Garlic Lamb Chops

SERVES 4 / PREP: 10 MINUTES + 1 HOUR, 30 MINUTES MARINATING TIME
COOK: 8 MINUTES + 5 MINUTES RESTING TIME

Fine-dining restaurants specialize in creating dishes that seem wonderfully elaborate but, in reality, are delicious because they're made from high-quality ingredients. When these lamb chops come off your grill and you savor your first juicy bite, four-star restaurant cuisine will come to mind. If you do not have a grill, broil the chops for 5 minutes per side in the oven.

3 garlic cloves, peeled

1 tablespoon chopped fresh thyme

1 teaspoon chopped fresh rosemary leaves

1 teaspoon lemon zest

Pinch sea salt

Pinch freshly ground black pepper

¼ cup olive oil

8 (4-ounce) lamb chops, about ¾-inch thick and trimmed of fat

1. In a blender, combine the garlic, thyme, rosemary, lemon zest, sea salt, and pepper. Pulse until finely chopped.

2. Add the olive oil. Pulse until a thick paste forms.

3. In a medium bowl, combine the lamb chops and garlic paste. With clean hands, rub the paste all over the chops. Cover and refrigerate for 1 hour to marinate.

4. Remove the bowl from the refrigerator. Let the chops sit for about 30 minutes to come to room temperature.

5. Preheat the grill (or broiler) to medium.

6. Grill the chops for about 4 minutes per side for medium-rare, or until your desired doneness.

7. Let the chops rest for 5 minutes and serve 2 per person.

(Per Serving) Calories: 431; Total Fat: 25g; Saturated Fat: 6g; Carbohydrates: 2g; Fiber: 0g; Protein: 48g

Lamb Burgers with Mint

SERVES 4 / PREP: 15 MINUTES + 1 HOUR CHILLING TIME / COOK: 20 MINUTES

Serve these moist herb-infused burgers on plump, gluten-free sesame seed–topped hamburger buns. Top with tangy tzatziki sauce, thick tomato slices, and a handful of crisp, shredded lettuce to finish. You can also serve them on a bed of lettuce or form them into small appetizer-size meatballs, depending on your preference. No matter how you serve them, take care to cook them until just a hint of pink remains in the center so they remain juicy and tender.

1 pound lean ground lamb

1 large egg

½ sweet onion, finely chopped

¼ cup chopped fresh mint

¼ cup chopped fresh parsley

1 teaspoon minced garlic

¼ teaspoon sea salt

¼ teaspoon freshly ground black pepper

1. In a large bowl, mix together the lamb, egg, onion, mint, parsley, garlic, sea salt, and pepper.

2. Shape the mixture into 4 patties about ¾ inch thick. Place the burgers on a plate, cover with plastic wrap, and refrigerate for 1 hour.

3. Preheat the grill (or broiler) to medium.

4. Grill the burgers, turning once halfway through, for about 20 minutes, or until they are just cooked through. Serve.

PHASE 1: (Per Serving) Calories: 240; Total Fat: 10g; Saturated Fat: 3g; Carbohydrates: 2g; Fiber: 0g; Protein: 34g

PHASE 2: (Per Serving) Calories: 267; Total Fat: 12g; Saturated Fat: 5g; Carbohydrates: 4g; Fiber: 1g; Protein: 35g

PHASE 2 TIP: Serve the burgers on gluten-free buns topped with a tablespoon of Homemade Coconut Yogurt (page 120).

Beef-Stuffed Tomatoes

SERVES 4 / PREP: 15 MINUTES + 30 MINUTES DRAINING TIME / COOK: 40 MINUTES

Stuffed baked vegetables are fun to make and fun to eat because the container that holds the tasty filling is edible, too. The tomatoes should not be too ripe, because you do not want them to be difficult to hollow out without tearing the sides or to split when baked. Use beefsteak tomatoes that are deep and wide for the best results.

Olive oil, for the baking dish

4 large firm tomatoes, tops sliced off and pulp removed

Sea salt

1 pound lean ground beef

½ sweet onion, chopped

1 teaspoon minced garlic

1 red bell pepper, chopped

1 cup cooked red lentils

2 tablespoons chopped fresh parsley

2 tablespoons chopped fresh basil

Freshly ground black pepper

1. Preheat the oven to 350°F. Lightly coat an 8-by-8-inch baking dish with olive oil and set aside.

2. Sprinkle the tomato shells with sea salt and place them upside down on paper towels to drain for 30 minutes.

3. While the tomatoes are draining, place a large skillet over medium heat. Sauté the ground beef for about 6 minutes, crumbling, until no pink remains.

4. Add the onion, garlic, and bell pepper. Sauté for about 3 minutes, or until the vegetables are tender.

5. Remove from the heat and stir in the lentils, parsley, and basil. Season the filling with sea salt and black pepper.

6. Place the tomato shells right-side up in the prepared dish. Spoon equal amounts of filling into the tomatoes. Place in the preheated oven and bake for about 30 minutes, or until tender and the filling is warm.

(Per Serving) Calories: 430; Total Fat: 8g; Saturated Fat: 3g; Carbohydrates: 39g; Fiber: 18g; Protein: 49g

Grilled Sirloin with Sautéed Bell Peppers

SERVES 4 / PREP: 15 MINUTES / COOK: 30 MINUTES

Omega-3 fatty acids are important on a candida-free diet because they can reduce inflammation, which can help support a healthy gut. If you want to increase the omega-3 fatty acids in beef, opt for grass-fed beef. It also has a higher vitamin E content, which helps boost the immune system.

1 tablespoon olive oil, divided

1 pound boneless top sirloin steak, about 1 inch thick, trimmed of visible fat

Sea salt

Freshly ground black pepper

2 teaspoons minced garlic

2 red bell peppers, sliced thin

1 yellow bell pepper, sliced thin

1 scallion, chopped

1 cup stemmed shredded Swiss chard

1 teaspoon chopped thyme

1. Preheat the grill (or broiler) to medium.

2. With 1 teaspoon of the olive oil, lightly brush the steak on both sides. Season the meat lightly with sea salt and black pepper. Grill the steak for about 5 minutes per side for medium (160°F), or until your desired doneness. Transfer the steak to a cutting board and let it rest for at least 10 minutes.

3. While the steak is resting, place a large skillet over medium heat and add the remaining 2 teaspoons of olive oil. Sauté the garlic for about 2 minutes, or until fragrant.

4. Add the red bell peppers, yellow bell pepper, and scallion. Sauté for about 5 minutes, or until tender.

5. Add the Swiss chard and thyme. Toss the mixture with tongs for about 2 minutes, or until the greens wilt. Season the mixture with sea salt and black pepper.

6. Slice the steak across the grain into at least 16 thin strips and transfer the meat to 4 plates. Top the steak with the bell pepper mixture and serve.

PHASE 1: (Per Serving) Calories: 356; Total Fat: 21g; Saturated Fat: 8g; Carbohydrates: 6g; Fiber: 2g; Protein: 33g

PHASE 2: (Per Serving) Calories: 358; Total Fat: 21g; Saturated Fat: 8g; Carbohydrates: 6g; Fiber: 2g; Protein: 33g

PHASE 2 TIP: Add 1 tablespoon of raw apple cider vinegar to the sautéed bell pepper mixture before serving.

PHASE 1 **PHASE 2**

Classic Pot Roast

SERVES 4 / PREP: 10 MINUTES / COOK: 6 HOURS, 15 MINUTES

Depending on how you like roast beef, a slow cooker is a nice alternative to the oven. The steps are the same and, if your slow cooker is set to high, the timing will also be identical. If you are in Phase 3 and want a thicker gravy than the jus produced here, remove the meat and vegetables from the pot and whisk 1 tablespoon of arrowroot into the accumulated juices before serving.

2 sweet potatoes, peeled and cut into 2-inch chunks

2 carrots, peeled and cut into 1-inch chunks

2 celery stalks, cut into 2-inch pieces

1 sweet onion, cut into 8 wedges

3 garlic cloves, slightly smashed

2 bay leaves

2 fresh rosemary sprigs, lightly crushed

½ cup Beef Bone Broth (page 54), or purchased beef broth

1 teaspoon olive oil

1 (1½-pound) beef chuck roast

¼ teaspoon sea salt

¼ teaspoon freshly ground black pepper

1. Preheat the oven to 300°F.

2. In a roasting pan with a lid, combine the sweet potatoes, carrots, celery, onion, garlic, bay leaves, rosemary sprigs, and beef broth.

3. Place a medium skillet over medium heat and add the olive oil. Season the beef lightly all over with sea salt and pepper.

4. Brown the roast on all sides in the hot skillet. Then, place the roast on top of the vegetables in the roasting pan. Cover the pan and place it in the preheated oven. Roast the meat for about 6 hours or until very tender.

5. Arrange the roast and vegetables on a serving plate. Remove and discard the bay leaves and rosemary sprigs.

6. Pour any accumulated juices from the roasting pan over the meat and serve.

PHASE 1: (Per Serving) Calories: 482; Total Fat: 16g; Saturated Fat: 5g; Carbohydrates: 23g; Fiber: 4g; Protein: 59g

PHASE 2: (Per Serving) Calories: 484; Total Fat: 16g; Saturated Fat: 5g; Carbohydrates: 23g; Fiber: 4g; Protein: 59g

PHASE 2 TIP: Add 2 tablespoons of raw apple cider vinegar to the broth in the roasting pan to give the meat a more complex flavor.

Beef Goulash

SERVES 4 / PREP: 15 MINUTES / COOK: 35 MINUTES

Paprika is the defining spice in this Hungarian dish, providing color and a spicy kick to the sauce. Stirring the paprika into the beef drippings and olive oil while off the heat ensures that the flavor releases without the chance of burning the spice. If you cannot find smoked paprika, try hot or sweet paprika instead.

1 (1-pound) beef shoulder roast, cut into 1-inch pieces

1 tablespoon arrowroot flour

Sea salt

1 tablespoon olive oil

1 sweet onion, chopped

2 teaspoons minced garlic

1½ tablespoons smoked paprika

2 large tomatoes, chopped

1 red bell pepper, diced

1 cup Beef Bone Broth (page 54) or purchased beef broth

½ cup Homemade Coconut Yogurt (page 120)

1 scallion, chopped

Brown rice or gluten-free noodles, for serving

1. In a medium bowl, toss the beef chunks with the arrowroot flour and salt until the meat is coated.

2. Place a large skillet over medium heat and add the olive oil. Brown the meat for about 6 minutes, in batches, until all of the beef is browned. Return the meat to the skillet.

3. Add the onion and garlic. Sauté for 3 minutes. Remove the skillet from the heat.

4. Stir in the paprika so the spice coats the meat and vegetables. Place the skillet back over medium heat. Add the tomatoes and red bell pepper. Sauté for 5 minutes.

5. Stir in the beef broth and bring the sauce to a simmer. Reduce the heat to low. Simmer for about 10 minutes, or until the meat is tender.

6. Stir in the yogurt. Top with the scallion and serve the goulash over brown rice or gluten-free noodles.

(Per Serving) Calories: 269; Total Fat: 14g; Saturated Fat: 5g; Carbohydrates: 14g; Fiber: 4g; Protein: 24g

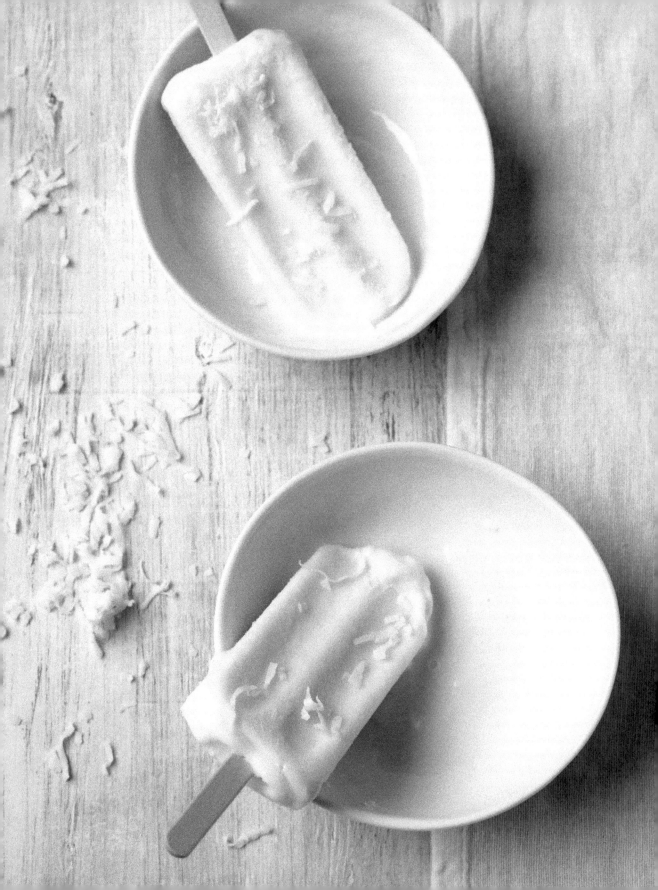

Chapter 8

Desserts

Coconut Ice Pops

MAKES 6 ICE POPS / PREP: 10 MINUTES / FREEZING: 4 HOURS

Nothing beats a cool, sweet treat on a sweltering summer day. So, why limit ice pops to snacks when they make elegant desserts after a spicy or barbecued meal? Coconut milk comes in many forms, from a thin, milk-like product in a carton to a thick version in a can with an exotic label. For this recipe, use the coconut milk that comes in a can and has a thick cream layer on top when you open the can. This ensures your ice pops will be decadent and rich.

2 cups canned full-fat unsweetened coconut milk (2 [14-ounce] cans)

½ cup shredded unsweetened coconut

2 tablespoons granulated stevia

1 teaspoon alcohol-free vanilla extract

1. In a large bowl, whisk the coconut milk to emulsify. It will be separated when you pour it from the can. Measure out the 2 cups you need and reserve the rest for another use.

2. Add the coconut, stevia, and vanilla and whisk together until blended.

3. Pour the mixture into 6 ice pop molds. Freeze for about 4 hours, or until firm.

PHASE 1: (Per Serving, 1 ice pop) Calories: 278; Total Fat: 27g; Saturated Fat: 25g; Carbohydrates: 6g; Fiber: 1g; Protein: 2g

PHASE 2: (Per Serving, 1 ice pop) Calories: 299; Total Fat: 28g; Saturated Fat: 25g; Carbohydrates: 11g; Fiber: 2g; Protein: 3g

PHASE 2 TIP: Stir 1 cup of fresh blueberries into the coconut mixture before pouring into the molds.

Panna Cotta

SERVES 4 / PREP: 20 MINUTES + 2 HOURS CHILLING TIME / COOK: 5 MINUTES

This stripped-down version of traditional panna cotta takes very little time to put together and has a lovely and pronounced strawberry flavor. Other fruit, such as raspberries, mangos, peaches, or even tart kiwi, can work, but strawberries create a delightful pastel-pink dessert. Locally grown, in-season strawberries have the best flavor.

1 tablespoon unflavored gelatin

2 cups unsweetened almond milk, at room temperature

½ cup raw honey

1 cup puréed strawberries

1. In a medium saucepan, sprinkle the gelatin on the almond milk and let sit for 10 minutes.

2. Place the saucepan over medium heat. Stir the mixture for about 5 minutes, or until the gelatin dissolves. Do not let it boil.

3. Whisk in the honey and strawberries. Remove from the heat and cool for 10 minutes.

4. Pour the panna cotta mixture evenly among 4 (6-ounce) ramekins. Refrigerate for 2 hours or more to chill. Serve.

(Per Serving) Calories: 166; Total Fat: 2g; Saturated Fat: 0g; Carbohydrates: 39g; Fiber: 1g; Protein: 2g

COOKING TIP: Fresh strawberries can be puréed easily, but simmering them with 2 tablespoons of water for about 5 minutes intensifies the color. After puréeing the berries, strain out the seeds to create a smooth texture.

Coconut–Brown Rice Pudding

SERVES 6 / PREP: 10 MINUTES / COOK: 1 HOUR + 30 MINUTES RESTING TIME

Rice pudding is as homey as the warm lights of home after a long trip. Brown rice adds a pleasing chewy texture and the almonds, a satisfying crunch. If you like pudding thinner in consistency, add a few extra tablespoons of coconut milk to your bowl before eating this comforting dessert.

4 cups unsweetened coconut milk

1½ cups short-grain brown rice

½ cup raw honey

1 teaspoon alcohol-free vanilla extract

½ teaspoon ground cinnamon

¼ teaspoon sea salt

Pinch ground nutmeg

½ cup sliced almonds

1. In a large saucepan set over medium heat, stir together the coconut milk, brown rice, honey, vanilla, cinnamon, sea salt, and nutmeg. Bring to a boil. Reduce the heat to low and simmer for about 1 hour, stirring frequently, or until the rice is very tender and the liquid is almost entirely absorbed.

2. Remove the pudding from the heat and let it rest for 30 minutes.

3. Spoon into small dessert bowls or ramekins, top with the almonds, and serve.

(Per Serving) Calories: 334; Total Fat: 9g; Saturated Fat: 3g; Carbohydrates: 65g; Fiber: 5g; Protein: 5g

Lime Mousse

SERVES 4 / PREP: 15 MINUTES + 4 HOURS CHILLING TIME

Coconut cream, the thick layer at the top of the canned coconut milk, is a versatile ingredient that adds richness to a recipe, adds moisture to baked products, and whips up as fluffy as heavy cream. If you have never tried whipped chilled coconut cream, the texture and volume might take you by surprise. This simple dessert relies on careful folding to retain as much volume as possible. Use a rubber spatula and take your time.

2 (14-ounce) cans full-fat unsweetened coconut milk, refrigerated for at least 4 hours

¼ cup freshly squeezed lime juice

2 teaspoons lime zest

¼ cup granulated stevia

1. Scoop out the thick coconut fat layer at the top into a large bowl. Save the liquid at the bottom of the can for another recipe.

2. With an electric hand mixer, beat the coconut fat for about 10 minutes, or until very thick and fluffy.

3. Add the lime juice, lime zest, and stevia. Beat to combine.

4. Refrigerate for 4 hours. Spoon the mousse into 4 small serving bowls and serve.

(Per Serving) Calories: 232; Total Fat: 24g; Saturated Fat: 21g; Carbohydrates: 6g; Fiber: 2g; Protein: 2g

Oatmeal Crème Brûlée

SERVES 4 / PREP: 15 MINUTES / COOK: 40 MINUTES + 30 MINUTES COOLING TIME

You will not be wielding a handheld propane torch to caramelize sugar into a crisp topping for this dessert because the top gets golden and crispy in the oven. Leftovers would make a lovely breakfast the next day, although leftovers are unlikely.

Coconut oil, for the baking dish

1½ cups unsweetened coconut milk

1 large egg

1 teaspoon alcohol-free vanilla extract

1 cup gluten-free rolled oats

4 teaspoons granulated stevia

¼ teaspoon ground cinnamon

⅛ teaspoon sea salt

1. Preheat the oven to 350°F. Lightly coat an 8-by-8-inch baking dish with coconut oil.

2. In a large bowl, whisk together the coconut milk, egg, and vanilla. Stir in the oats, stevia, cinnamon, and sea salt.

3. Evenly spread the mixture into the prepared dish and place it in the preheated oven. Bake for about 40 minutes, or until the edges are firm.

4. Remove the dish from the oven to a wire rack. Cool for 30 minutes before serving.

PHASE 1: (Per Serving) Calories: 306; Total Fat: 24g; Saturated Fat: 20g; Carbohydrates: 19g; Fiber: 4g; Protein: 6g

PHASE 2: (Per Serving) Calories: 342; Total Fat: 27g; Saturated Fat: 21g; Carbohydrates: 22g; Fiber: 4g; Protein: 7g

PHASE 2 TIP: Serve each portion topped with 1 tablespoon of Homemade Coconut Yogurt (page 120).

Easy Avocado Pudding

SERVES 4 / PREP: 10 MINUTES

Lime juice adds a fresh citrus tang to this pudding and ensures that the avocados do not oxidize and turn an unpleasant brownish color. You can adjust the amount of stevia in the recipe because the finished pudding is not overly sweet. Make sure your avocados are very ripe before blending them or the texture of the dish will be grainy rather than velvety.

3 avocados, peeled and pitted

¾ cup freshly squeezed lime juice

2 teaspoons granulated stevia

1 teaspoon alcohol-free vanilla extract

⅛ teaspoon sea salt

1. In a food processor (or blender), combine the avocados, lime juice, stevia, vanilla, and sea salt. Purée until very smooth and creamy.

2. Scoop the pudding into 4 small dishes and serve.

PHASE 1: (Per Serving) Calories: 313; Total Fat: 29g; Saturated Fat: 6g; Carbohydrates: 14g; Fiber: 10g; Protein: 3g

PHASE 2: (Per Serving) Calories: 345; Total Fat: 30g; Saturated Fat: 6g; Carbohydrates: 21g; Fiber: 14g; Protein: 4g

PHASE 2 TIP: Top each portion with ½ cup of fresh raspberries.

Elegant Almond-Sesame Cookies

MAKES 12 COOKIES / PREP: 20 MINUTES / COOK: 10 MINUTES

It is best to store these golden treats up high and someplace inconvenient because they are completely addictive. The cookie is melt-in-your-mouth tender and the toasty sesame seed coating is delectable.

1¼ cups almond flour

¼ cup granulated stevia

½ teaspoon baking soda

¼ teaspoon sea salt

½ cup tahini
(sesame paste)

1 tablespoon melted
coconut oil

2 teaspoons alcohol-free
vanilla extract

½ cup sesame seeds

1. Preheat the oven to 350°F. Line a baking sheet with parchment paper and set aside.

2. In a large bowl, stir together the almond flour, stevia, baking soda, and sea salt until well mixed.

3. In a small bowl, stir together the tahini, coconut oil, and vanilla.

4. Stir the tahini mixture into the almond mixture until blended.

5. In a separate small bowl, add the sesame seeds and place it next to the bowl with the cookie dough.

6. Form the dough into 1-inch balls and then roll them in the sesame seeds. Place the cookies on the prepared sheet and flatten them slightly with the base of a heavy glass. Place the cookies into the preheated oven and bake for about 10 minutes, or until they are light brown.

7. Remove them from the oven and transfer the cookies to rack to cool completely. Refrigerate the cookies in an airtight container for up to 1 week or freeze them for up to 1 month.

(Per Serving) Calories: 181; Total Fat: 16g; Saturated Fat: 3g; Carbohydrates: 6g; Fiber: 3g; Protein: 3g

Citrus-Vanilla Cake

SERVES 8 / PREP: 10 MINUTES / COOK: 30 MINUTES

If you need a birthday or event cake that is candida-free diet approved, whip up this recipe and your guests will never know it isn't an old family favorite. This cake has a fine, tender crumb and intense lemon flavor, which can be enhanced with fresh berries either as a topping or in the batter. Make sure the almond flour is very fine rather than a coarse meal to achieve the cake's light texture.

Coconut oil, for coating the pan

½ cup arrowroot flour, plus more for the pan

4 large eggs, separated

1 tablespoon lemon zest

¼ cup raw honey

1 teaspoon alcohol-free vanilla extract

1 cup fine almond flour

1 teaspoon baking powder

¼ teaspoon ground nutmeg

Pinch sea salt

1. Preheat the oven to 350°F. Lightly coat a 9-inch round cake pan with coconut oil. Dust it with arrowroot flour and set aside.

2. In a large bowl, whisk together the egg yolks, lemon zest, honey, and vanilla. Stir in the almond flour, the ½ cup of the arrowroot flour, baking powder, and nutmeg.

3. In a large, dry, clean bowl, beat the egg whites and sea salt with an electric hand mixer (with clean, dry beaters) until soft peaks form. Gently fold the beaten egg whites into the cake batter, retaining as much volume as possible.

4. Spoon the batter into the prepared cake pan and place it into the preheated oven. Bake for about 30 minutes, or until the top springs back when pressed lightly.

5. Remove from the oven and cool completely on a wire rack.

(Per Serving) Calories: 166; Total Fat: 10g; Saturated Fat: 1g; Carbohydrates: 13g; Fiber: 2g; Protein: 5g

INGREDIENT TIP: Scrub lemons very well to remove surface wax and any lingering pesticides on the skin before zesting the fruit. Even organic lemons should be washed well to remove contaminants from the shipping and handling of the fruit.

Angel Food Cake

SERVES 12 / PREP: 20 MINUTES / COOK: 40 MINUTES

Cream of tartar is often the stabilizer of choice when whipping egg whites into a fluffy, stiff meringue, but this ingredient can promote yeast overgrowth. Lemon juice is also acidic, so it acts similarly to the cream of tartar and is an easy substitution: Use 1 teaspoon of lemon juice for every egg white in the recipe and you will not even miss the cream of tartar.

12 large egg whites, at room temperature

4 tablespoons freshly squeezed lemon juice

2 tablespoons granulated stevia

1 teaspoon alcohol-free vanilla extract

1 cup fine almond meal

1. Preheat the oven to 350°F.

2. In a large, clean, dry bowl, beat the egg whites with an electric hand mixer (that has clean and dry beaters) on medium until frothy.

3. Add the lemon juice. Beat the whites on high speed until stiff peaks form. Reduce the speed to low.

4. Stir in the stevia and vanilla. Gently fold the almond meal into the beaten egg whites.

5. Spoon the batter into an angel food cake pan and smooth the top with a spatula. Place the cake in the preheated oven and bake for about 40 minutes, or until the top is golden and springs back when touched lightly.

6. Remove the cake from the oven, turn the pan upside down, and cool completely.

PHASE 1: (Per Serving) Calories: 72; Total Fat: 5g; Saturated Fat: 0g; Carbohydrates: 2g; Fiber: 1g; Protein: 6g

PHASE 2: (Per Serving) Calories: 80; Total Fat: 5g; Saturated Fat: 0g; Carbohydrates: 5g; Fiber: 1g; Protein: 6g

PHASE 2 TIP: Serve each slice with ¼ cup of pitted cherries.

Mixed Fruit Crumble

SERVES 6 / PREP: 15 MINUTES / COOK: 30 MINUTES

Following a special diet to alleviate a medical condition can make you feel deprived, especially when it comes to desserts. If crumble, crisp, buckle, and brown Betty were favorite desserts before starting this diet, you will be pleased that this recipe is as good as any sugar-laden recipe you might have made in the past. The delicate, crispy topping and delicious fruit filling are absolutely gorgeous in a serving bowl and will tempt you to have a second serving, if there is any left.

¼ cup coconut oil, plus more for the baking dish

1 cup fresh blueberries

1 cup fresh raspberries

1 apple, peeled, cored, and chopped

1 peach, pitted and chopped

2 tablespoons chia seeds

1 tablespoon freshly squeezed lemon juice

2 teaspoons granulated stevia, divided

1 cup gluten-free rolled oats

½ cup chopped walnuts

¼ cup almond flour

½ teaspoon ground cinnamon

¼ teaspoon ground nutmeg

1. Preheat the oven to 325°F. Lightly coat an 8-by-8-inch baking dish with coconut oil.

2. In a large bowl, toss together the blueberries, raspberries, apple, peach, chia seeds, lemon juice, and 1 teaspoon of the stevia. Spread the fruit mixture evenly in the prepared dish.

3. In a small bowl, stir together the oats, walnuts, almond flour, the remaining 1 teaspoon of stevia, the cinnamon, and nutmeg.

4. Add the ¼ cup of coconut oil to the oat mixture. With clean fingertips, blend the coconut oil into the oat mixture until the mix resembles coarse crumbs. Sprinkle the topping over the fruit.

5. Place the fruit crumble in the preheated oven and bake for about 30 minutes, or until the filling is bubbly and the topping is golden brown.

6. Remove from the oven and cool.

(Per Serving) Calories: 288; Total Fat: 20g; Saturated Fat: 8g; Carbohydrates: 26g; Fiber: 6g; Protein: 8g

INGREDIENT TIP: Chia seeds make an effective thickener for the filling so the juices seeping from the fruit turn into a thick sauce rather than creating a soggy topping. You can also try arrowroot powder if chia seeds are not available.

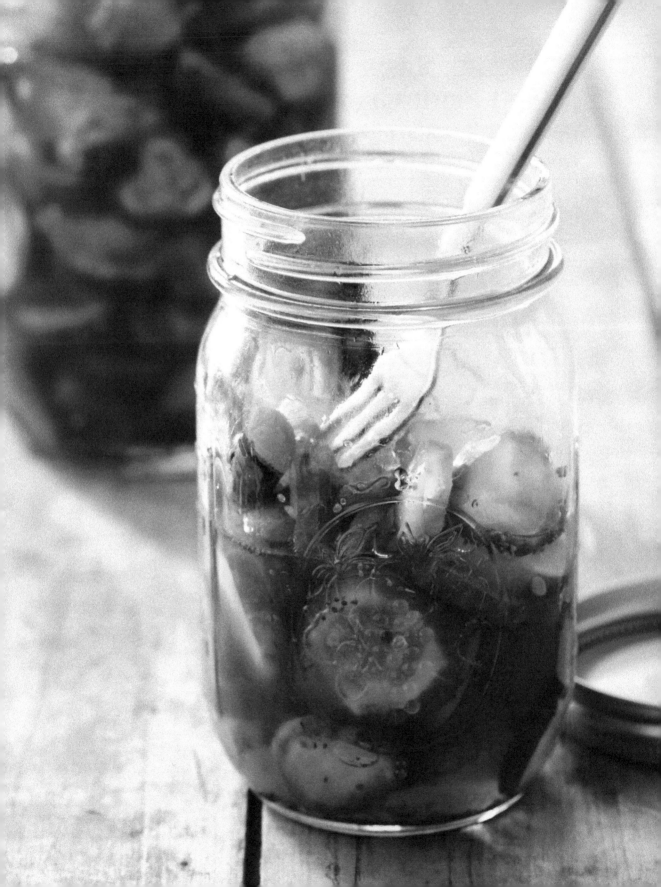

Chapter 9

Fermented Foods

Fermented foods can enhance many recipes in this book and your candida-free diet in general. Often used as condiments or toppings, these foods also have intense flavors and add healthy probiotics to the meal. The recipes are so easy to make—especially in large quantities—that you might wonder why your pantry and refrigerator aren't full of jars packed with pretty fermented products. Most fermented foods have a strong taste, so add them in small amounts.

Homemade Coconut Yogurt

MAKES 4 CUPS / PREP: 30 MINUTES + 12 HOURS FERMENTING TIME

Making yogurt might seem like it ranks right up there with churning your own butter, but the process for yogurt is actually quite easy and requires very little physical effort. The kefir provides the beneficial yeast necessary to culture the coconut milk into a tangy yogurt. You can find kefir in most supermarkets or health food stores.

2 cups unsweetened coconut milk

¼ cup coconut kefir

¼ cup coconut water

3 tablespoons freshly squeezed lemon juice

1. Add the coconut milk, coconut kefir, coconut water, and lemon juice and process until smooth and creamy, about 10 minutes.

2. Transfer the yogurt mixture to a large jar or glass bowl and cover tightly with a fine-mesh cheesecloth.

3. Let the yogurt mixture sit at room temperature for at least 12 hours to ferment and thicken.

4. When thickened, stir the yogurt and transfer it to an airtight storage container.

5. Keep refrigerated for up to 1 week.

(Per Serving) Calories: 209; Total Fat: 19g; Saturated Fat: 17g; Carbohydrates: 10g; Fiber: 5g; Protein: 2g

Sauerkraut

MAKES 1 QUART / PREP: 30 MINUTES + 7 TO 10 DAYS FERMENTING TIME

Sauerkraut is German for "sour cabbage," although this vegetable preparation could have been found over 2,000 years ago in China using rice wine instead of the salt found in the German version. This tangy dish can boost digestive health, stimulate the immune system, and support cardiovascular health. The process of fermenting the cabbage does not use heat, which could kill the beneficial bacteria that makes fermentation possible.

1 head green cabbage, finely shredded, with 4 large outer leaves reserved

2 tablespoons sea salt

Distilled water, as needed

1. Sterilize 2 (1-quart) jars and lids by placing them in a pot and filling the pot with water so the jars are covered by about 2 inches. Bring to a boil over high heat and boil for 10 minutes. With clean tongs, remove them and set aside to cool.

2. In a large bowl, toss together the cabbage and salt, scrunching it with your hands until liquid comes out. Continue to massage the cabbage for about 10 minutes, until it is watery.

3. In the sterilized jars, pack the cabbage tightly. Distribute the leftover liquid from the bowl evenly between the jars.

4. Pack 2 cabbage leaves into each jar, on top of the shredded cabbage, and add distilled water if the liquid does not cover the shredded cabbage completely.

5. Cover the mouth of the jars with fine-mesh cheesecloth and secure with a rubber band. Place the jars in a cool, dark place. Ferment the sauerkraut for 7 to 10 days.

6. When the sauerkraut is tangy enough for your taste, top tightly with the clean lids, and refrigerate for up to 3 months.

(Per Serving) Calories: 22; Total Fat: 0g; Saturated Fat: 0g; Carbohydrates: 5g; Fiber: 2g; Protein: 1g

Kimchi

MAKES 2 QUARTS / PREP: 20 MINUTES + 3 DAYS FERMENTING TIME

Kimchi is Korean in origin and references to it can be found in Korean poetry that is over 3,000 years old. Preserving vegetables using salt is one of the ways people still received nutrients and minerals during winter months when fresh produce was scarce.

1 head napa cabbage, cut into 2-inch pieces

6 tablespoons plus ½ teaspoon sea salt, divided

Cold water, as needed

2 scallions, cut into 2-inch pieces

1 cup sliced daikon radish

1 (6-inch) piece peeled ginger, sliced

¼ cup fish sauce

1 tablespoon minced garlic

¼ teaspoon cayenne pepper

2 teaspoons granulated sugar

1. In a large bowl, combine the cabbage with 6 tablespoons of the sea salt. Toss to coat.

2. Add enough cold water to cover the cabbage completely and then cover the bowl with plastic wrap. Let the cabbage sit at room temperature for 12 hours. Then, drain and rinse the cabbage with cold water.

3. With clean hands, squeeze the excess liquid from the cabbage and transfer it to another large bowl.

4. Add the scallions, daikon radish, ginger, fish sauce, garlic, cayenne pepper, sugar, and remaining ½ teaspoon of sea salt. Stir until the ingredients are evenly combined.

5. Sterilize 2 (1-quart) jars and their lids by placing them in a pot and filling the pot with water so the jars are covered by about 2 inches. Bring the water to a boil over high heat. Boil the jars for 10 minutes. Then, with clean tongs, carefully remove and set aside to cool.

6. Pack each sterilized jar tightly with the cabbage mixture and seal with the lids. Let the jars sit in a cool, dark place for 24 hours and then open the jars to let the pressure escape.

7. Reseal the jars and refrigerate the kimchi for at least 48 hours before eating it.

8. Keep refrigerated for up to 1 month.

(Per Serving) Calories: 18; Total Fat: 0g; Saturated Fat: 0g; Carbohydrates: 3g; Fiber: 1g; Protein: 1g

Dill Pickles

**MAKES 2 QUARTS / PREP: 15 MINUTES + 2 WEEKS TO FERMENTING TIME
COOK: 10 MINUTES**

You can use this basic pickle recipe with any type of vegetable or an assortment of vegetables, like cauliflower, green beans, beets, carrots, or asparagus. The salt quantity is not high in this brine compared to other traditional preparations, but it can still be a concern if hypertension is an issue for you. Pickles should be eaten in moderation if you are following a low-sodium diet.

20 pickling cucumbers

4 garlic cloves, smashed, divided

4 fresh dill sprigs, divided

½ teaspoon black peppercorns, divided

4 cups distilled water

¼ cup sea salt

1. Sterilize 2 (1-quart) jars and lids by placing them in a pot and filling the pot with water so the jars are covered by about 2 inches. Bring to a boil over high heat and boil for 10 minutes. With clean tongs, remove the jars and set them aside to cool.

2. Pack each jar half full with cucumbers. Then add 1 garlic clove, 1 dill sprig, and a few peppercorns.

3. Top the jars with the remaining cucumbers along with 1 garlic clove, 1 dill sprig, and a few peppercorns.

4. In a small saucepan set over medium heat, combine water and sea salt, stirring until the salt is dissolved. Remove the saucepan from the heat.

5. Pour the salt brine into the 2 jars, evenly dividing it. Add more distilled water, if necessary, so the cucumbers are covered by at least 1 inch. Seal the jars and place them in a cool, dark place for 2 weeks.

6. Check the jars daily to see if pressure is building up. If the center of the lid can't be pressed down, unscrew the lid just enough to open it.

7. After 2 weeks, refrigerate and eat the pickles within 2 months.

(Per Serving, 2 pickles) Calories: 18; Total Fat: 0g; Saturated Fat: 0g; Carbohydrates: 4g; Fiber: 2g; Protein: 1g

Lacto-Fermented Lemons

MAKES 1 QUART / PREP: 15 MINUTES + 2 WEEKS FERMENTING TIME

North African food features preserved lemon, often including spices, unlike this simple version. The pulp of these lemons can be used for sauces, stews, porridges, and desserts. The pith and peel are intensely lemony and add complexity to any dish. Lacto-fermented lemons are also a wonderful source of probiotics, which are crucial for candida management.

2 pounds lemons

3 tablespoons sea salt, divided

1. Scrub the lemons to remove any wax applied for transport. Trim the ends off the lemons, taking care not to cut into the flesh of the fruit. Cut them into quarters almost all the way through, keeping them attached at the stem end. They will look like a four-petal flower.

2. Sprinkle the cut lemon edges with sea salt.

3. In a clean 1-quart mason jar, pack 2 lemons.

4. Sprinkle the lemons with sea salt and then use a wooden spoon to mash them until they release their juice. Repeat this process of packing, salting, and mashing until all the lemons are packed into the jar and the liquid is just above the top of the lemons. Cover the jar with a tight lid.

5. Let the jar sit at room temperature for 2 weeks to ferment. If the lid is very tight, open it slightly, daily, to release excess pressure.

6. After 2 weeks, refrigerate the preserved lemons for up to 4 months.

(Per Serving) Calories: 16; Total Fat: 0g; Saturated Fat: 0g; Carbohydrates: 5g; Fiber: 2g; Protein: 1g

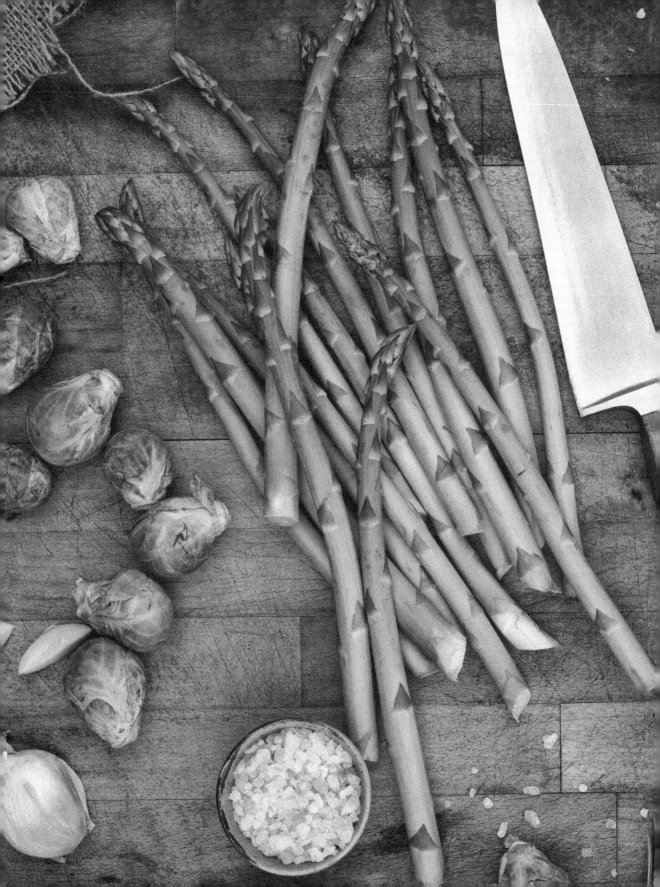

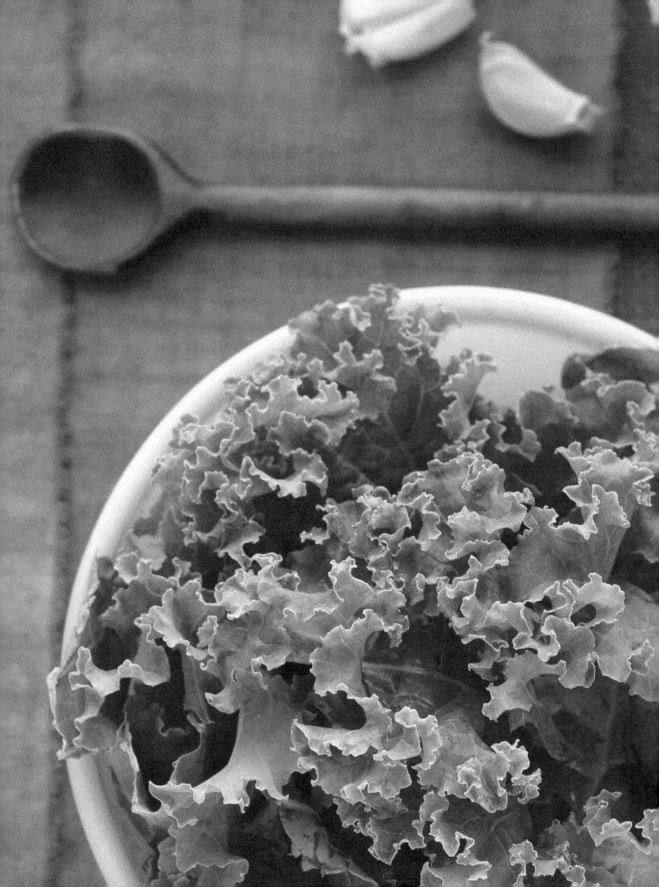

Measurement Conversions

Volume Equivalents	U.S. Standard	U.S. Standard (ounces)	Metric (approximate)
Liquid	2 tablespoons	1 fl. oz.	30 mL
	¼ cup	2 fl. oz.	60 mL
	½ cup	4 fl. oz.	120 mL
	1 cup	8 fl. oz.	240 mL
	1½ cups	12 fl. oz.	355 mL
	2 cups or 1 pint	16 fl. oz.	475 mL
	4 cups or 1 quart	32 fl. oz.	1 L
	1 gallon	128 fl. oz.	4 L
Dry	⅛ teaspoon	—	0.5 mL
	¼ teaspoon	—	1 mL
	½ teaspoon	—	2 mL
	¾ teaspoon	—	4 mL
	1 teaspoon	—	5 mL
	1 tablespoon	—	15 mL
	¼ cup	—	59 mL
	⅓ cup	—	79 mL
	½ cup	—	118 mL
	⅔ cup	—	156 mL
	¾ cup	—	177 mL
	1 cup	—	235 mL
	2 cups or 1 pint	—	475 mL
	3 cups	—	700 mL
	4 cups or 1 quart	—	1 L
	½ gallon	—	2 L
	1 gallon	—	4 L

Oven Temperatures

Fahrenheit	Celsius (approximate)
250°F	120°C
300°F	150°C
325°F	165°C
350°F	180°C
375°F	190°C
400°F	200°C
425°F	220°C
450°F	230°C

Weight Equivalents

U.S. Standard	Metric (approximate)
½ ounce	15 g
1 ounce	30 g
2 ounces	60 g
4 ounces	115 g
8 ounces	225 g
12 ounces	340 g
16 ounces or 1 pound	455 g

Resources

Specialty Ingredients

Amazon.com
Bob's Red Mill: BobsRedMill.com
Navitas Naturals: NavitasNaturals.com
Organic Matters: OMFoods.com
Prana: PranaSnacks.com
Rancho Vignola: RanchoVignola.com
Thrive Market: ThriveMarket.com
Whole Foods Market: WholeFoodsMarket.com

Supplements

Body Ecology: BodyEcology.com/all-products.html
Flora Health: FloraHealth.com
GAPS Diet: Shop.GAPSDiet.com
Garden of Life: GardenOfLife.com
Genuine Health: GenuineHealth.com
Harmonic Arts: HarmonicaArts.ca
The Honest Company: Honest.com
iHerb: iHerb.com
Natural Factors: NaturalFactors.com
Webber Naturals: WebberNaturals.com

Websites

BodyEcology.com
BodyEcology.com/quiz-php/ (for candida questionnaire)
RickiHeller.com
TheCandidaDiet.com
YeastConnection.com/pdf/yeastfullsurv.pdf (for candida questionnaire)

References

Ben-Ami, Ronen, et al. "Antibiotic Exposure as a Risk Factor for Fluconazole-Resistant Candida Bloodstream Infection." *Antimicrobial Agents and Chemotherapy* 56, no. 5 (2012): 2,518–2,523. doi:10.1128/AAC.05947-11.

Body Ecology. "PMS and Candida Overgrowth: The Dangers of Estrogen Dominance." January 17, 2020. Accessed December 8, 2020. BodyEcology.com/articles/pms -and-candida-overgrowth-the-dangers-of-estrogen-dominance.

Brown, Kirsty, Daniella Decoffe, Erin Molcan, and Deanna L. Gibson. "Diet-Induced Dysbiosis of the Intestinal Microbiota and the Effects on Immunity and Disease." *Nutrients* 4, no. 8 (August 21, 2012): 1095–119. doi:10.3390/nu4081095.

Campbell, Andrew W. "Autoimmunity and the Gut." *Autoimmune Diseases* 2014 (May 13, 2014): 152428. doi:10.1155/2014/152428.

Casqueiro, J., J. Casqueiro, and A. Cresio. "Infections in Patients with Diabetes Mellitus: A Review of Pathogenesis." *Indian Journal of Endocrinology and Metabolism* 16, Supp. 1 (March 2012): 27. doi:10.4103/2230-8210.94253.

Centers for Disease Control and Prevention. "Antifungal Resistance." November 20, 2020. Accessed December 8, 2020. CDC.gov/fungal/antifungal-resistance .html#eleven.

_____. "Invasive Candidiasis Statistics." April 20, 2020. Accessed December 8, 2020. CDC.gov/fungal/diseases/candidiasis/invasive/statistics.html.

Chattopadhyay, Sanchari, Utpal Raychaudhuri, and Runu Chakraborty. "Artificial Sweeteners—A Review." *Journal of Food Science and Technology* 51, no. 4 (2011): 611–21.

Childs, Caroline, Philip Calder, and Elizabeth Miles. "Diet and Immune Function." *Nutrients* 11, no. 8 (2019): 1933. doi:10.3390/nu11081933.

Dean, Carolyn. "Candida—Yeast Gone Wild." N.E.E.D.S. Accessed December 8, 2020. Needs.com/product/NDNL-0704-01/a_Candida.

_____. "Probiotics—Yeast Gone Wild." N.E.E.D.S. Accessed December 8, 2020. Needs .com/product/NDNL-0704-01/a_Probiotics.

De Leon, Ella, Scott Jacober, Jack Sobel, and Betsy Foxman. "Prevalence and Risk Factors for Vaginal Candida Colonization in Women with Type 1 and Type 2 Diabetes." *BMC Infectious Diseases* 2, no. 1 (2002).

Donders, Gilbert G., Gert Bellen, and Werner Mendling. "Management of Recurrent Vulvo-Vaginal Candidosis as a Chronic Illness." *Gynecologic and Obstetric Investigation* 70, no. 4 (2010): 306–21. doi:10.1159/000314022.

Fichorova, Raina N., et al. "The Contribution of Cervicovaginal Infections to the Immunomodulatory Effects of Hormonal Contraception." *MBio* 6, no. 5 (2015). doi:10.1128/mBio.00221-15.

Gates, Donna. "Honey, Sugar, Molasses, Agave, Stevia, and Other Natural Sweeteners: Which Are Actually Good for You?" June 28, 2007. Accessed December 8, 2020. BodyEcology.com/articles/which_are_good_sweeteners-php.

Gates, Donna, and Linda Schatz. *The Body Ecology Diet: Recovering Your Health and Rebuilding Your Immunity.* Carlsbad, California: Hay House, 2011.

Gross, Lee, Li, Earl Ford, and Simin Lu. "Increased Consumption of Refined Carbohydrates and the Epidemic of Type 2 Diabetes in the United States: An Ecologic Assessment." *American Journal of Clinical Nutrition* 79, no. 5 (2004): 774–79.

Heller, Ricki, and Andrea Nakayama. *Living Candida-free: 100 Recipes and a 3-Stage Program to Restore Your Health and Vitality.* Philadelphia, PA: Da Capo Press, 2015.

Kühbacher, Andreas, Anke Burger-Kentischer, and Steffen Rupp. "Interaction of Candida Species with the Skin." *Microorganisms* 5, no. 2 (June 2017): 32. doi:10.3390/microorganisms5020032.

Kumamoto, Carol A. "Inflammation and Gastrointestinal Candida Colonization." *Current Opinion in Microbiology* 14, no. 4 (August 2011): 386–391. doi: 10.1016/j.mib.2011.07.015.

Lennerz, Belinda, et al. "Effects of Dietary Glycemic Index on Brain Regions Related to Reward and Craving in Men." *American Journal of Clinical Nutrition* 98, no. 3 (September 2013): 641–647. doi:10.3945/ajcn.113.064113.

Levin, Warren M., and Fran Gare. *Beyond the Yeast Connection: A How-to Guide to Curing Candida and Other Yeast-Related Conditions.* Laguna Beach, CA: Basic Health Publications, 2013.

Lipski, Elizabeth. *Digestive Wellness*. 3rd ed. New York, NY: McGraw-Hill, 2005.

Mavor, A. L., S. Thewes, and B. Hube. "Systemic Fungal Infections Caused by Candida Species: Epidemiology, Infection Process, and Virulence Attributes." *Current Drug Targets* 6, no. 8 (2005): 863–74.

McCombs, Jeffrey. *The Everything Candida Diet Book: Improve Your Immunity by Restoring Your Body's Natural Balance*. Avon, MA: F + W Media, 2014.

Mu, Qinghui, Jay Kirby, Christopher M. Reilly, and Xin M. Luo. "Leaky Gut as a Danger Signal for Autoimmune Diseases." *Front Immunol* 8 (May 23, 2017): 598. doi:10.3389/fimmu.2017.00598.

Murray, Michael, and Joseph Pizzorno. *Encyclopedia of Natural Medicine*. 2nd ed. New York, NY: Three Rivers Press, 1998.

Pattani, Reena, Valerie Palda, Stephen Hwang, and Prakeshkumar Shah. "Probiotics for the Prevention of Antibiotic-Associated Diarrhea and Clostridium Difficile Infection among Hospitalized Patients: Systematic Review and Meta-Analysis." *Open Medicine* 7, no. 2 (2013).

Pollan, Michael. "Some of My Best Friends Are Germs." *The New York Times*. May 18, 2013. December 8, 2020. NewYorkTimes.com/2013/05/19/magazine/say-hello-to-the-100-trillion-bacteria-that-make-up-your-microbiome.html.

R, Arya and Naureen B. Rafiq. "Candidiasis." StatPearls [Internet], U.S. National Library of Medicine. November 20, 2020. NCBI.NLM.NIH.gov/books/NBK560624.

Resta, Silvia C. "Effects of Probiotics and Commensals on Intestinal Epithelial Physiology: Implications for Nutrient Handling." *The Journal of Physiology* 587, Pt 17 (September 2009): 4,169–174. Published online July 13, 2009. doi:10.1113/jphysiol.2009.176370.

Richards, Lisa. "Candida and Oral Contraceptives." The Candida Diet. May 10, 2019. Accessed September 9, 2015. TheCandidaDiet.com/candida-oral-contraceptives.

_____. "How Are Hangovers Related to Candida?" The Candida Diet. April 8, 2019. Accessed December 8, 2020. TheCandidaDiet.com/acetaldehyde-and-candida.

_____. "How Does Candida Change Your Gut Flora After Antibiotics?" The Candida Diet. February 20, 2019. Accessed December 8, 2020. TheCandidaDiet.com/candida-changes-gut-flora-after-antibiotics.

_____. "Should You Take Probiotics and Antifungals Together?" The Candida Diet. January 13, 2017. Accessed December 8, 2020. TheCandidaDiet.com/taking -probiotics-and-antifungals-together.

_____. "When Should You Take Probiotics?" The Candida Diet. October 20, 2019. Accessed December 8, 2020. TheCandidaDiet.com/when-take-probiotics.htm.

Stoppler, Melissa Conrad. "Candidiasis (Yeast Infection, Candida)—When Should You Call a Doctor for a Yeast Infection?" EMedicineHealth, October 10, 2019. Accessed December 8, 2020. eMedicineHealth.com/candidiasis_yeast_infection /article_em.htm.

Taubes, Gary. "Is Sugar Toxic?" *The New York Times Magazine.* April 16, 2011. Accessed September 9, 2015. NYTimes.com/2011/04/17/magazine/mag -17Sugar-t.html?_r=0.

The European Food Information Council. "The Role of Gut Microorganisms in Human Health." October 1, 2013. Accessed December 8, 2020. EUFIC.org/en /healthy-living/article/the-role-of-gut-microorganisms-in-human-health.

University of Michigan."Vaginal Yeast Infections More Common When Using Contraceptives or Spermicides, or Participating in Receptive Oral Sex." *Michigan News.* December 11, 2006. Accessed December 8, 2020. News.UMich.edu/vaginal -yeast-infections-more-common-when-using-contraceptives-or-spermicides-or -participating-in-receptive-oral-sex.

World Health Organization. "Antimicrobial Resistance." October 13, 2020. Accessed December 8, 2020. www.WHO.int/health-topics/antimicrobial-resistance.

Yan, Lei, Chunhui Yang, and Jianguo Tang. "Disruption of the Intestinal Mucosal Barrier in Candida Albicans Infections." *Microbiological Research* 168, no. 7 (2013): 389–395. doi:10.1016/j.micres.2013.02.008.

Index

Printed in the USA
CPSIA information can be obtained
at www.ICGtesting.com
LVHW061055080124
768205LV00002B/6